Chelation Therapy

Other Books by Morton Walker, D.P.M.

DMSO ('76 Press, 1981)

Rebounding Aerobics (National Institute of Reboundology and Health, 1981)

How Not to Have a Heart Attack (Franklin Watts, 1980)

Nutrients to Age without Senility (Keats Publishing, 1980)

The Complete Book of Birth (Simon & Schuster, 1979)

Total Health: The Holistic Alternative to Traditional Medicine that Stresses Preventive Care, Nutrition and Treatment of the Whole Person (Everest House, 1979)

Advertising and Promoting the Professional Practice (Hawthorn Books, 1979, Second Edition, revised 1981 and released by Freelance Communications and the Third Edition, revised 1982 and released by Macmillan Publishing Co. in the late spring 1982)

Orthomolecular Nutrition: New Lifestyle for Super Good Health (Keats Publishing, 1978)

Help Your Mate Lose Weight (Jove Publications, 1978)

Sport Diving: The Instructional Guide to Skin and Scuba (Contemporary Books, 1977)

The Medical School Admission Adviser (Hawthorn Books, 1976, revised and released in 1981 by Elsevier-Dutton with the new title *How to Get into Medical School)*

Think and Grow Thin (Arco Publishing, 1973 reprinted in 1978 by Arco under the new title *Lose Weight/Gain Health/Live Longer)*

Your Guide to Foot Health (Follett Publishing, 1964, reprinted by Arco Publishing in 1972)

To be published in the spring 1982:

Medical Practice Management Desk Book (Prentice-Hall)

Chelation Therapy

How To Prevent Or Reverse Hardening Of The Arteries

Dr. Morton Walker

M. EVANS & COMPANY, INC. / NEW YORK, N.Y. 10017

Dedication

To the members of the American Academy of Medical Preventics, who are following the precepts of the Hippocratic Oath in its true meaning

ISBN 0-87131-365-0

LC 81-69734

M. Evans and Company, Inc.
216 East 49 Street
New York, New York 10017

Manufactured in the United States of America

9 8 7 6 5 4

Table of Contents

Preface

In early spring four years ago, when I was preparing the proposal for a book on techniques to reverse hardening of the arteries, one of the scientists I consulted, Elliot M. Goldwag, Ph.D., said to be sure and include chelation therapy. "What's that?" I asked.

Perhaps like you, I was newly exposed to the therapeutic wonders of EDTA chelation. My investigations have since convinced me that chelation therapy has the ability to save the lives of more than a million Americans annually.

The steady but ubiquitous hardening of our arteries drains vitality from the cells and tissues of the body. It disables and kills by blocking blood circulation to the heart, brain, internal organs, or limbs. It narrows arterial channels, reduces blood flow, cuts off oxygen, suffocates blood vessels themselves, and prevents nourishment from reaching the anatomical areas these starved arteries supply. Yet, treatment taken with an intravenous infusion of EDTA chelation reverses each of these pathological processes. My four years of research since I learned of the therapy, interviewing more than one hundred physicians who give the injections and several hundred patients who have taken them, has proven beyond question that medical science has a potent tool to stop the diseases derived from the degeneration of our arteries.

Every second person who dies in this country each year is killed, directly or indirectly, by degeneration of the arteries. But the absolute reversal of the clogging mechanism in arteries can be accomplished without surgery, without pain, and without radiation. The chemotherapy used is nontoxic, nutritional, medicinal, comfortable, and involves physician participation. It does ask you to change your lifestyle, as an essential part of altering the degeneration process within the arteries.

People in North America, Europe, and other parts of the industrialized world do not have to die prematurely anymore from hardening of the arteries. This book tells you how to reverse the process.

This book can save your life. I hope you will use it!

Morton Walker, D.P.M.
Stamford, Connecticut

Acknowledgments

Hundreds of contributors assisted me in bringing you the information in this book: chelation therapy patients who told me their stories, the physicians who administered their treatments, the patients' loved ones who filled in objective details, their friends and neighbors who verified the facts I uncovered, and medical librarians who dug into archives.

In gathering research material, I had a lot of other help, too. I want to acknowledge the diligent efforts of Garry F. Gordon, M.D. of Sacramento, California, Chairman of the Board of Trustees and immediate past president of the American Academy of Medical Preventics, Inc., who supplied me with a great deal of clinical journal material, case histories, and who checked the entire manuscript for accuracy. Dr. Gordon remained a continuous source of inspiration, even when the subject of chelation therapy kept getting rejected by publishers.

I thank Beverly Newkirk of The Committee for Freedom of Choice in Cancer Therapy, Inc.

I appreciate the input of Harold W. Harper, M.D. of Los Angeles, also a former president of the Academy, who set up appointments with colleagues and provided me with his own experiences. I thank Bruce W. Halstead, M.D. of Colton, California, who is current president of AAMP; Yiwen Y. Tang, M.D. of San Francisco; and Charles H. Farr, M.D., Ph.D. of Norman, Oklahoma, all of whom furnished case histories, illustrative materials, and shared their own experiences with chelation techniques. Warren M. Levin, M.D. of New York City unselfishly granted me much of his time; and, Norman E. Clarke, M.D., "the grandfather of EDTA chelation," provided a scientific treatise on atherosclerosis he had prepared for a medical meeting.

Of everyone, Joan Walker, my loving and patient spouse, deserves the most thanks because she suffered through the periodic publisher rejections with me. She had as much investment in time — having lost my attention during its writing — from my involvement with this book. Furthermore, she was my built-in editor who helped cull the vast amount of medical material into the more manageable manuscript that finally evolved. Without my wife's assistance, I couldn't have turned in the final script for copyediting to Chip Wood.

The more I researched, the greater was my realization that this story was the most important piece of medical journalism I had ever undertaken. In uncovering facts for you, Joan and I have learned how to preserve our own lives and health, too.

Morton Walker, D.P.M.

Foreword

I currently serve as Chairman of the Board of Trustees and immediate past president of the American Academy of Medical Preventics, Inc., a group of traditionally trained physicians who have broken from precedent and offer the controversial, but highly beneficial, chelation therapy. Dr. Morton Walker has described the intravenous technique of chelation with the disodium salt of ethylene diamine tetraacetic acid (EDTA) in this carefully researched, well-documented, and entirely correct book. He has taken an exceedingly technical medical subject and provided us with an entertaining, clear, and easy-reading explanation of what chelation therapy is, how it works in the body, the method of administration, how much it costs, the time it takes to administer, what happens from its administration, why people need it and want it, who are the beneficiaries, when it is given, and a thousand other answers to questions potential patients may have.

Dr. Walker has also documented the opposition to chelation therapy and presented its history — the whole story. There are many ramifications to this opposition, something the author dug into so that he provides us more than just the medical marvels of a treatment. He has, in fact, shown some failures in our modern system of health care delivery.

Today's over-utilized, over-publicized heart surgery is a good example of our failure to deal effectively with causes of hardening of the arteries. Instead, we spend millions of dollars treating the results of occlusive arterial disease. Excellent medical studies have shown that most bypass heart patients do no better (and many do *worse*) than those who receive much safer drug therapy at a mere fraction of the cost. Yet even drug therapy does not address itself to the basic causes of heart disease. In spite of well-controlled studies demonstrating the shortcomings of experimental bypass surgery for coronary heart disease, the use of this surgical procedure by American hospitals and physicians is increasing so rapidly that it could become the largest single item in our entire Federal budget by 1988.

Change is obviously needed and long overdue. Rather than concentrating on some new methods of funding this failing health care system, we must first redirect our thoughts and efforts to develop and practice true preventive medicine concepts as an integral part of a new health delivery system. Indeed, this must be a national priority item.

We all seem to need more motivation to follow a healthier lifestyle long before our health has deteriorated to the point that it becomes obvious to us or to our physician. Fortuitously, technological developments at this time have resulted in the growth of new, highly sophisticated, yet entirely painless methods of "non-invasive" testing of our circulatory status. These techniques will allow your physician to determine accurately how much circulatory impairment you have before recognizable symptoms, such as leg cramps, appear. Such testing provides us with an important form of feedback information which can help motivate us to incorporate important changes in how we live into our daily routine. Such actions performed not for a day, not for a month, but for a lifetime will demonstrably improve our health and slow down or even prevent (reverse?) our hardening of the arteries.

Too bad that almost all major medical progress has initially encountered broad skepticism and even open hostility from the leaders of the orthodox medical community. After all, their basic beliefs are usually challenged by any significant breakthrough in medical knowledge. This negative response is largely due to the by now well-documented 30 to 50 year time lag that occurs between the initial discovery of a major new concept and its later broad general acceptance by the medical world. The history of penicillin, vitamin C, iodine, niacin, and even the acceptance of modern surgical antisepsis are all classic examples that demonstrate this unfortunate fact.

Today this delay may be even further aggravated by government regulations and interference intended to control the *costs* of medical care and administered with typical bureaucratic inefficiency through gigantic, virtually uncontrollable government agencies, best exemplified by the Food and Drug Administration of the Federal Government. Their resistance to change is assisted by the usual skepticism of "orthodox" members of medical societies and even medical boards, which are usually under the direct control of organized medicine. These impediments to progress are further aided by the physicians' reluctance to be innovative, due to the constant threat of malpractice suits as well as by the pressure of peer-group opinion. In addition, the economic interests of health insurance companies causes them to place additional barriers in the path of medical progress. We now have government sanctioned peer review committees and other quasi-governmental health planning agencies that, collectively, threaten to halt invaluable medical advances. Without innovation, there is no progress.

Of course, this is all done in the name of the "consumer," who is told he needs this protection as he is not able to decide on health care matters for himself. Why? The agencies warn the consumer might be subject to some form of quackery or even fraud.

Unfortunately, no one explains to the consumer that in these efforts to "protect" him, there can be more real danger to his health than from all the health quacks in the world. He may finally be denied all innovative treatments until they become "approved" at some distant time — which may be years after he is dead. He might have spent the remaining funds in his estate trying to help himself, even trying unproved therapies. So it doesn't appear that the bureaucrats are really operating in the consumer's best interest after all. Who will protect us from a government grown too big and too powerful?

It is my belief that the facts and information contained in *Chelation Therapy: How To Prevent or Reverse Hardening of the Arteries* will motivate citizens of the industrialized West to maintain their own good health, along with maintaining their medical freedom of choice, before it becomes truly too late for either. This means that significant medical concepts such as "informed consent," and "benefit-to-risk ratios" must become generally discussed by all of us. Americans and other westerners should think for themselves so that we can once again return to that unique climate of medical freedom that allowed the United States to become one of the great world leaders in medical progress.

Dr. Morton Walker has done all of us a service by investing his skill as a medical journalist in this subject of chelation therapy. Admittedly, it is an extremely controversial subject in medicine and because of that, the author has had a difficult time in getting this book published.

Use of the information in *Chelation Therapy: How To Prevent or Reverse Hardening of the Arteries* can save lives — yours, mine, and the lives of a million-and-a-quarter other Americans who die each year from the effects of occlusive arterial disease. We have the potential to live the full span of man's life — 120 years — if we take care of our health. This book will help you approach that lifespan with a quality of living immeasureably improved over anything you have now. All that's needed is that you act upon the information written here.

Garry F. Gordon, M.D., Chairman of the Board of Trustees and immediate past president, the American Academy of Medical Preventics, Inc., Sacramento, California

Chapter One

You Can Reverse
Hardening of the Arteries

From the womb of darkness and the cocoon of indifference is emerging a form of treatment that will eventually be added to the armamentarium of the alert and concerned physician.

— Richard E. Welch, M.D.
Let's Live, April 1976

New Life for Old Arteries

While golfing under the Southern California sun in December 1971, George W. Frankel, M.D., of Long Beach, California, Chief of Otolaryngology at two hospitals and staff ear, nose and throat specialist at three others, was seized by severe chest pains. His golfing partners returned him to the club house, and after resting Dr. Frankel visited his cardiologist.

Following electrocardiograms and treadmill tests, a coronary angiogram was performed at the hospital. Dr. Frankel was told by the cardiologist and a chest surgeon that his angiogram revealed obstructing plaques in the left main coronary artery. They recommended a triple coronary artery bypass. This operation must be done as soon as possible, the specialists said, in order to avoid coronary occlusion and, possibly, sudden death.

Coronary artery bypass surgery involves the removal of one of the major veins from the patient's thigh and its use to bypass the arteries feeding the heart that are being occluded. Such a surgery entails several serious hazards. There is a 10 to 15 percent possibility of a heart attack while on the operating table; there can be later aggravated deterioration of the arteries bypassed; there is a 20 to 30 percent possibility of occlusion of the new graft within two years; and, there is the possibility of the reappearance, after a few years, of similar chest pains, with little or no chance of relief by additional surgery. Although the mortality of this operation at this writing is approximately 5 to 12 percent, the morbidity, better known as the *complications*, still exist in another 10 to 15 percent of the cases done. That is, one patient in fifteen will die *during the operation*; one in seven will suffer complications *after* the surgery.

Physicians experience fear of life-threatening procedures as does anyone else, and this ear, nose and throat specialist was no exception. Dr. Frankel was not anxious to face major surgery on his heart, but there seemed to be no alternative. Consequently, he did agree, and the surgery was scheduled to be performed in a few days. Then fate changed his course. Seven units of blood were needed for standby during the operation, but the Red Cross could not obtain this blood until after the Christmas and New Year holidays. His heart surgery was therefore rescheduled for two weeks later.

During his wait, Dr. Frankel discussed his condition with many of his colleagues and friends. One friend, whom Dr. Frankel described to me as "a very dear colleague who went to medical school with me, interned with me, and later became a prominent internist in New York," told of another individual with a similar condition. That person went through a treatment called *chelation*, a medical therapy that apparently reduced the amount of calcium in the obstructing plaques of the coronary arteries and reduced the amount of calcium in other areas of the vascular system.

Dr. Frankel, eager to try any logical, safe and painless avenue that might avoid the very real potential of death offered by heart surgery, began to search for clinical literature on the subject at the Los Angeles County Medical Association Library. He was amazed to find numerous medical journal articles on chelation therapy, a treatment he had never heard of before. After careful study of these many references, the patient ventured on what he hoped to be a journey to save his life. He entered an Alabama hospital which was run by H. Ray Evers, M.D.

"I saw people come in with diabetic ulcerative lesions and gangrenous lesions that cleared up in a matter of ten or twelve days, and I could not believe my eyes," said Dr. Frankel. "I saw one patient who was admitted after being told elsewhere that his leg would have to be amputated because of gangrene, and, daily, after chelation therapy, I watched with my mouth agape, as the leg came back to normal. I acted as a sort of assistant to Dr. Evers by making rounds with him every day. He was a very determined man who worked twenty of every twenty-four hours."

There was something else that Dr. Frankel could hardly believe. Prior to treatment, anginal pains had seared his chest when he walked only ten or twelve steps. After he received only ten chelations, the pain disappeared entirely. He went on to take twenty chelation treatments in Alabama and felt 75 percent better than before. He decided to put off having the heart surgery indefinitely. In the event he needed surgery later, the patient knew that his chance of survival was considerably enhanced by the remarkable improvement he experienced from his chelation treatments.

The physician-patient has since given himself eighty-eight more chelations at home — with the help of a nurse-anesthetist for the intravenous injections — a total of 108 treatments in all. "And I want to tell you that I have not had an angina since early January, 1972," says Dr. Frankel. "I carry a full work load. I do approximately ten to fifteen surgeries every week, and these are microsurgeries of the ear. I carry a full practice. I play golf. I swim twenty laps in my pool every day, and I cannot speak with any but the greatest praise for the men who are attempting to make chelation an accepted form of therapy."

* * * * *

After enjoying an outing in very hot weather during the fall of 1975, Roland C. Hohnbaum, D.C., then fifty-four years old, a chiropractic doctor in Richmond, California, noticed that an ulcer had developed on his left foot. Such an ulcer was highly dangerous for Dr. Hohnbaum, since he is a long-term diabetic. Even with knowledge of the ramifications of diabetic ulcers, the chiropractor told himself "this can't happen to me. I'm different!" But he was not different, and the gangrenous course of arteriosclerosis complicated by diabetes began its insidious creep from his toes upward.

"It grew worse and worse, and finally I was forced down and was flat on my back for about two months," said Dr. Hohnbaum. "I had an internist at the Alta Bates Hospital in Berkeley, California in whom I had a lot of confidence. He took care of my case in the beginning but then he became frightened, too, saying that I'd have to go to the hospital because I was going to lose my toes."

Also quite frightened himself, Dr. Hohnbaum knew it was time to make some major decisions. He rejected the amputation because of gangrene, since he knew that a decision to operate just *started* at the toes. Gangrene is known to spread, slowly and steadily, and eventually may require amputation below the knee, above the knee, or even at mid-thigh. Besides, the combination of hardening of the arteries and diabetes were by now showing effects in his other foot, too. It possibly meant having both feet cut off.

Because he refused hospitalization and surgery, Dr. Hohnbaum was denied further treatment by both his internist and the consulting vascular surgeon. Afflicted as he was, the patient had to engage in his own self-help program at home by bringing in dietary factors and anything else he could use to improve his health. He prayed that his condition might begin to show some improvement.

"I finally found out about Dr. Tang with the chelation therapy," the chiropractor said, while tears formed in his eyes, "and this was a life-saver for me. I don't think that I can say any more than that I — I have feet under me now."

When Dr. Hohnbaum visited Yiwen Y. Tang, M.D., F.A.B.F.P. of San Francisco, he arrived on crutches and in pain. "The patient was in immediate need of amputation of his two legs below the knee," Dr. Tang told me. "His life was in imminent danger. He could bear nothing on his feet — not hosiery — certainly not shoes." Dr. Tang supplied me with photographs which depict the condition of Dr. Hohnbaum's feet. After careful diagnostic studies, Dr. Tang began Dr. Hohnbaum on chelation treatments.

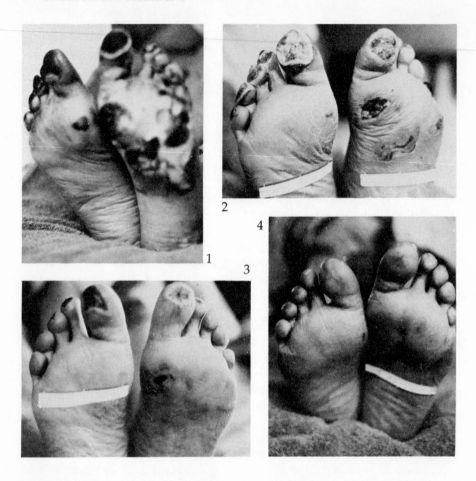

Photograph 1 shows the feet of Roland C. Hohnbaum, D.C., two days before his scheduled operation for amputation because of diabetic gangrene and ulcerations. He could bear nothing on his feet, not even hosiery, because of the pain. Following standard medical procedure, both legs would have been cut off below the knees. After just one week of chelation therapy, however *(Photograph 2)*, the gangrene has been reversed and the ulcerated areas are beginning to heal. Two months after the last of fifteen chelation treatments *(Photograph 3)*, the diabetic gangrene was eliminated and Dr. Hohnbaum wore shoes and returned to work full time. Two months later *(Photograph 4)*, all ulcerations have disappeared and Dr. Hohnbaum's feet are completely normal.

"The pre-chelation tests also indicated clogging of my carotid artery, making me a prime target for stroke," said Roland Hohnbaum.

Within a week of having the first treatment the patient could put on socks. By January 1976, two months after the last of fifteen chelations, he wore shoes and returned to work full time. The chiropractor is now completely healed with no evidence of anything having happened to his feet.

"Post-chelation tests show my carotid artery now clear of occlusion," Dr. Hohnbaum told me. "There is no doubt that the atherosclerosis which accompanied my diabetes has been abated."

Dr. Hohnbaum's case and a dozen others like his have changed medical thinking in this country about diabetic gangrene. The condition had previously been diagnosed as irreversible, but diabetic ulcers and gangrene now can be cured by chelation therapy.

Dr. Hohnbaum added a postscript to his story. He said, "I am still haunted by the flat statement made to me by a vascular surgeon whom I had met after my feet were all healed. Upon seeing the photographs of my gangrenous feet, the surgeon said, 'If you had been my patient and your feet looked like these pictures, there is no question — I would have amputated!' "

* * * * *

During the Thanksgiving holidays in 1973, Lester I. Tavel, D.O. of Houston, Texas made a visit to his friend, Harold W. Harper, M.D. of Los Angeles, California. Dr. Tavel complained of no particular health problem, but as doctors will do for each other, Dr. Harper performed a physical examination on his colleague. At the examination's conclusion, Dr. Harper advised his friend to take chelation treatment as a precautionary measure against occlusial artery disease. Then Dr. Harper gave Dr. Tavel chelation materials to use for self-treatment at home.

"But being an osteopathic physician, I made my own diagnosis and came to the decision that there was nothing wrong with me," confessed Dr. Tavel during our interview. "I did not give myself chelation therapy."

On March 31, 1974, Dr. Tavel suffered a heart attack, a paroxysmal atrial tachycardia with a pulse rate running at 200 beats per minute. It took three electric shocks of 25, 50, and 100 volts to cardiovert the victim back to a near-normal rate. An X-ray examination of his chest showed the patient's heart enlarged, filling practically the whole chest cavity. He remained in the intensive care unit of St. Luke's Hospital, Houston. Knowing of the risks that went with open-heart surgery, however, such an operation was not even considered by the osteopathic physician, his attending physicians, or his family.

As soon as Dr. Tavel could be moved, his wife flew with him to Dr. Harper's office in Los Angeles. Since her husband was unable to take more than three or four steps without experiencing tremendous shortness of breath, Mrs. Tavel pushed him in a wheel chair. The patient's ankles were swollen to the size of footballs.

Dr. Harper set up intravenous chelation in an apartment-hotel suite he had made ready for his friend. At the end of three weeks, in which he received fifteen treatments, the patient's heart began to return to its usual size. In another week, upon X-ray examination, it again appeared completely normal.

"You know, Los Angeles has a lot of streets with 45-degree inclines," Dr. Tavel later told me. "Well, by the time I had received thirty chelations in about six weeks, I was walking up the hill in front of my hotel. I walked up steps, too. My resting pulse rate was 84 beats per minute and by the time I reached the top of the hill, it increased to 110. Then it dropped back to 84 upon my resting within a minute afterwards."

"What Lester didn't know at the time,' said Dr. Harper, "is that his electrocardiogram (EKG) and enzyme studies indicated he had acute myocardial infarction (a local area of death) in the heart muscle. I began to administer therapy as soon as my emergency medical workup for him was over. After about the first five treatment days his shortness of breath began to go away. The edema (swelling) was down. He was able to eat again. His color changed from pasty white to something near his natural ruddiness.

"In the first week Lester was able to walk without being totally tired, as he had been when he arrived. His glucose tolerance test level had dropped to 15 milligrams percent (normal blood sugar is near 90) so I instituted a nutritional program during his treatment days," Dr. Harper revealed.

"I took a second X-ray series after about ten chelations. His heart size showed close to normal, but not quite. Lester's enzyme studies and blood sugar had returned to normal, though, and his EKG returned to normal within a two-week period." In fact, the EKG didn't even point to ischemia (inadequate circulation of blood).

"Follow-through at the end of thirty treatment days showed my patient's heart size comparable to the way it had been when I saw him the previous November. Comparison X-ray films attested to the heart sizes as being exactly the same. There were no fluid levels in his lungs — no congestion — no edema. Lester was able to go home at the end of six weeks," concluded Dr. Harper.

"I checked myself quite cautiously," Dr. Tavel added. "I ran a heck of a lot of BUNS (blood-urea-nitrogen tests for toxicity) and creatinines (urine tests) after I got home, and I didn't have any problems with those or any other toxic symptoms.

"I did notice many things about myself improve — my prior dyspnea (frequent rapid breathing) was relieved; my fatigue was relieved; my limbs were warmer," Dr. Tavel said. "I had a regrowth of hair on my legs, and I had an increased libido (sex drive) that my wife enjoyed. I gave myself ten more chelation treatments at home, and I've been taking six treatments a year since.

"About thirty days ago I had another chest X-ray that showed my heart size remaining normal. An independent group of cardiologists then evaluated my EKGs and rechecked about thirty-five of my laboratory tests, including all the heart enzyme tests and liver enzyme tests. All the diagnostic findings were back to normal as if I never had experienced a heart attack," Dr. Tavel assured me.

* * * * *

A triple coronary artery bypass was avoided; a gangrenous foot was not amputated, and the foot was restored to normal; a heart-attack victim rejects open-heart surgery, instead has a fluid enter his veins, and now says he is completely recovered. Can these stories possibly be true?

Every case history you will read about in this book is authentic. Every one you will read, I have double-checked for truth and accuracy. Dr. Tavel's story struck me as most dramatic. His heart problem had him closer to death than anyone ought to be, and still recover. I therefore took the opportunity to triple-check his story and sought out and interviewed a person who worked for Dr. Tavel at the time of his attack. I spoke with twenty-six-year-old Deborah Triche, a registered nurse employed by Dr. Tavel and his associate, Dr. John Mohney.

Nurse Triche retold the story of Dr. Tavel's heart attack that I have described. She said, "I was the technician who recorded Dr. Tavel's EKGs and submitted them to our cardiological EKG service. The heart doctors on the service read the recordings and computerize their reports. Each time a patient has an EKG taken it is compared to the one taken of him previously.

"Well, after Dr. Tavel's chelation therapy was completed, I asked one of the cardiologists about the comparisons between his pre-therapy and post-therapy EKGs. The cardiologist said, 'You know, Dr. Tavel's heart was severely damaged before the treatment, but now following chelation it shows no after-effects on the EKG at all.' I was amazed," said the nurse. Currently, chelation therapy is administered to patients requiring it in the Tavel-Mohney practice.

The History of Chelation Therapy

Chelation therapy is a well-recognized treatment for lead poisoning. It has been used to remove this poison metal from the bodies of children and other patients for over twenty-five years. The treatment has also been applied for reversal of hardening of the arteries with great success. Although not well recognized for anti-atherosclerotic purposes, chelation therapy is extensively documented in the medical literature, with at least 1,700 clinical and laboratory journal articles published in the English language. I have included a reference list of some of these articles in the footnotes and appendix. The articles provide additional supportive scientific evidence for the treatment's safety and efficacy.

Chelation therapy is not a new procedure. It was introduced into the United States in 1948, but it had been employed as a chemical medical treatment in Europe long before that. Presently, about one thousand physicians in this country offer the intravenous treatment. Approximately three million injections have been administered by them to around 120,000 patients.

The goal of the physician who gives chelation therapy is to restore adequate blood flow through his patient's occluded arteries and to relieve symptoms of arterial insufficiency anywhere in the body. This mode of therapy relieves the symptoms caused by atherosclerotic plaque that hardens and obstructs blood vessel walls. How it does this is the subject of considerable controversy and debate at this time. In this book, I shall present all of the known or currently held medical theory, established physiological or pathological facts, and the practical application of chelation therapy for atherosclerosis. My investigative medical reporting comes from clinical and laboratory journal articles, interviews with patients who experienced the treatment and physicians who give the injections, and my own investigations.

Chelation therapy administered to a patient is known to bind, or "chelate," divalent and trivalent metals in the human body. These metals have two or three combining bonds or valences. In the *concept of valence* in chemistry, the elements which do *not* combine with hydrogen — such as the metals — are said to have positive valence. Some of the metals, such as calcium, iron, zinc, lead, and mercury have two or three valences; they are *divalent* or *trivalent*.

The substance used to bring about chelation therapy is able to remove ionic calcium (a divalent metal) from the bloodstream and probably from the walls of the blood vessels, either directly or indirectly. This chemical substance is employed in the chelation intravenous injection. It carries dissolved liquid calcium from the bloodstream to the patient's kidneys and out of the body in the urine. The removed blood calcium is then replaced from the abnormal or unhealthy metastatic calcium deposits. These deposits act as a loose glue binding together the components of atherosclerotic plaque, so that the metastatic calcium leaves the plaque and ionizes in the blood. What happens to the plaque when it loses its glue? It breaks up and leaves the body.

Alterations in calcium and other divalent metals in the blood produce beneficial improvements in arterial enzyme function. They stabilize cellular membranes and enhance cellular function.

The ultimate effect of these physiological changes is an increased blood flow and an improvement in elasticity of hardened arteries. Additionally, there is probably a much-improved tissue perfusion through the capillaries, by decreasing the wall rigidity of red blood cells. Also, red blood cell aggregations are reversed. This decreases platelet "stickiness" by improving platelet membrane function. These net results appear to give "new life to old arteries."

A New Medical Alternative to Surgical Treatment
for Hardening of the Arteries

The basic chemical agent employed in chelation therapy, which I shall describe in the next chapter, has been shown by more than a hundred studies to be safe and effective against lead poisoning and other heavy metal contaminations. It is approved for this use by the Food and Drug Administration (FDA). The same mechanism that makes the drug a beneficial antidote against poisoning from lead makes it equally useful against excess serum calcium. Even so, chelation treatment to reverse hardening of the arteries is vigorously opposed by much of the American medical establishment.

My contention is that American medical consumers have the right to know about all their medical alternatives. Individual physicians have a legal and moral responsibility to inform patients of the various treatment choices available. This responsibility should be fulfilled regardless of whether the physician agrees or disagrees with the therapy.

As it stands now, a person who is suffering from hardening of the arteries generally receives incomplete information for this condition. The arteriosclerotic patient is not told of chelation therapy by his vascular surgeon — perhaps because most physicians don't know anything about the treatment themselves. In other instances physicians who think they know all about chelation may base their knowledge on hearsay and totally misleading information and not on any scientific study. They may, as a result, choose not to inform a patient who is contemplating bypass surgery or limb amputation about chelation therapy. Their reasons may be honorable. It might be that these physicians do not believe the treatment could really be effective. Legally, however, under prior court decisions, doctors must inform patients of *every* alternative — even if they personally reject one or more of the choices.

Chelation therapy is an alternative to painful, high-risk treatments, such as cardiovascular surgery with its high mortality rate, or to vasodilator drugs with their many side effects. Cardiovascular operations are prohibitively expensive and limited in their use, but these operations are terribly popular today. Surgery is restricted by the size of the blood vessels that can be operated upon. Tiny blood vessels cannot undergo surgical procedures, while in contrast chelation therapy can be used throughout the entire circulatory system.

In contemporary chelation treatment there have been *no known fatalities* as a result of its use. Conversely, death during or soon after bypass surgery is reported to range from 5 to 12 percent, depending on the experience of the heart surgeon and his staff. In surgical bypass the severity of the disease in the patient plays a part also. In fact, a study done by the National Institute of Health, which was reported to the medical community in March 1977, stated that no one should have a bypass operation except for the relief of intractable angina. Yet, nine out of ten of these same kinds of severe cardiac cases are reported entirely relieved of symptoms with chelation therapy. Obviously, the risk factor is almost eliminated.

That NIH report went on to say that general medical treatment rather than surgery was demonstrated to be safer and more effective for coronary arteriosclerosis cases.

The Status of Chelation Therapy in the United States

Legal problems connected with the main chelating agent that is used in this country are tied exclusively to economics. For instance, where the chelation agent once was accepted and recommended for the treatment of "occlusive vascular diseases" such as angina and was even paid for by health insurance companies, it appears now to have lost this official status as a result of a change in Federal regulations. The patents on the chelation drug expired in 1968. Because of this expiration, compliance to prove effectiveness under the new guidelines of Federal regulations would cost drug manufacturers millions of dollars. Drug companies cannot recover their money when the drug is no longer patentable. They therefore have no further interest in developing and marketing the product.

To attempt the licensing of a new drug, from scratch, in accordance with the safety and efficacy guidelines of the Food, Drug and Cosmetics Act as amended in 1962, and as currently enforced, involves up to ten years of trials and at least $14 million to $20 million in expenses. Such a great investment in time and money is required simply to get Food and Drug Administration approval. Then millions of dollars for advertising campaigns to physicians are necessary. Although not new, an unknown treatment like chelation therapy would need to be explained very carefully to practicing physicians in the United States.

It comes down to a matter of too many dollars and too much time required to bring chelation therapy to the American people. The plain and undeniable truth is that people are dying from atherosclerosis in part because of a lack of chelation therapy acceptance. The non-acceptance is caused by an absence of significant pharmaceutical industry investment potential.

Falling within the jurisdiction of the FDA are all those substances used in medical treatment which are construed to be either unlicensed new drugs or unsafe food additives. This includes safe and well-known substances such as aspirin, vitamin C, and nasal sprays, when used for a "new" purpose. The substance employed for chelation therapy is a safe food additive used in salad dressings (such as Hellmann's *Real* Mayonnaise®) and many other foods. It is listed on the GRAS list (generally recognized as safe by the FDA). Indeed, it is a licensed drug that is *not new* at all. Nevertheless, the FDA bans it from interstate shipment and sale anyway, if it is to be used for treatment of arteriosclerosis.

It is not banned if it is to be used for treatment of metallic poisoning. The agent is also used, and with U.S. Government sanction, for treatment of radioactive contamination. A story in the "Medicine" section in the March 21, 1977 issue of *Newsweek* magazine told of Harold McCluskey, a 64-year-old chemical operator, who had inhaled the largest recorded human dose of the isotope americium-241. His life was saved, sight restored, and radiation sickness prevented by the calcium salt of that same chelating agent which is banned from use against hardening of the arteries.[1]

The FDA ban is enforced even though the medication is the "drug of choice" for dealing with hardening of the arteries in other countries. For example, when atherosclerosis affects the legs of citizens of Czechoslovakia, this intravenous chelation injection treatment is given. The Czechs give full credit to American physicians for the discovery, but it remains bureaucratically suppressed in the United States.

The American Medical Association's department of medicine does not approve of chelation therapy for arteriosclerosis, either. Its status and worth for reversing hardening of the arteries "must be regarded with skepticism," says the AMA. And other doctors have referred in stronger terms to the various stories told by chelated patients. "Anecdoted medicine is bulls**t," says Alfred Soffer, M.D. of Chicago, a prominent internist, who is executive director of the American College of Chest Physicians. Dr. Soffer is a leading critic of chelation therapy.[2]

Most insurance companies today will not compensate holders of their health insurance policies for chelation treatment for arteriosclerosis. The patients are denied any reimbursement. The insurance industry has labeled the therapy "not usual, reasonable or customary" and generally refuses payment on those grounds, even if, because of chelation, the patient avoids ten of thousands of dollars in bills for bypass surgery (which the insurance companies *do* pay).

Chelation Certainly is "Reasonable" to Reynolds Hall

Although chelation is controversial, it certainly is "reasonable" to Reynolds Hall, age fifty-five, of Melbourne, Florida. It should be "usual and customary" also, he says, because the treatment for him generated a miracle.

Reynolds Hall is blind in his left eye as a result of a childhood accident. While shaving on the morning of June 23, 1973, he suddenly went blind in his right eye as well. "When my right eye went out, I couldn't see the mirror in front of me," Hall recalled to *Today* staff writer Howard Wolinsky.[3] (*Today* is a Gannett newspaper published in Brevard County, Florida.)

Hall said the vision in his right eye improved somewhat on its own during the time he was visiting physicians who specialize in eye and brain surgery. He was still considered legally blind when he was admitted to Brevard Hospital in Melbourne.

"After the testing was done, the docs said there was nothing they could do for me," Hall said.

Robert Rogers, M.D. of Melbourne, Hall's general practitioner, suggested chelation therapy since Hall suffers from arteriosclerosis. His hardening of the arteries had been so severe that the circulation of blood to his left leg had clogged completely and the leg was amputated in 1970.

Dr. Rogers suggested that the arteriosclerosis apparently was blocking arteries deep in Hall's head, causing the blindness to his remaining eye. The physician gave the patient intravenous chelation therapy while he was in the hospital in hopes of removing any blockage.

"After I took seven treatments, the miracle took place. I could see," said Hall. "I was looking across the room and about fifteen feet away I could read some tiny writing on the TV. It said 'Hospital Communications Systems.' I got real excited and called Dr. Rogers. When the doctor got to the hospital *he* couldn't even read the words. [The print was so small.]"

When an ophthalmologist checked his vision, it was found that Hall was 20/15 in his right eye — better than normal 20/20. In a letter that he wrote, another physician, Robert Sarnowski, M.D., a neurosurgeon in the Melbourne area, attested to the "dramatic" improvement in Hall's vision.

My Personal Note to the Reader

At this point in my writing I must interject a personal note about what you have read so far and what is to come. Usually, the conclusion that an objective observer draws, especially someone trained in science and medicine, like myself, is that Dr. Soffer's remark is correct. More often than not anecdotal medicine is nothing more than "buffalo dew." In the past I have believed that to be true. But what must an investigative medical journalist do when he is exposed to story after story and to one case history after another that reports potentially imminent death, blindness, amputation, paralysis and other problems among people, and upon visiting those people to check their stories, he sees them presently free of all signs of their former health problems. This has happened to me! About 200 individuals who were victims of hardening of the arteries are much changed. I have talked with them. They have become *former* victims. Now they are vibrant, productive, youthful looking, vigorous, full of zest for life, and they enthusiastically endorse chelation therapy as the cause of their prolonged good health.

I have checked most of what they said and turned up not a single untruth. Whether the scientific method accepts anecdotal evidence or not, the information about the effects of chelation therapy on hardening of the arteries deserves to be revealed. All persons whom I interviewed or corresponded with delivered their messages of recovery with ardor. They wish to share their sense of renewed health and well-being with others who are suffering or will suffer. Consequently, I decided to bring a number of their messages to you in this book. You may want the same thing that these people have found — freedom from hardening of the arteries.

Chapter Two

What the Chelation Process Is

There are no such things as incurables; there are only things for which man has not found a cure.

— Bernard Baruch, Address to the President's Committee on Employment of the Handicapped, May 1, 1954

"Physician, Heal Thyself"

His grandfather died at age fifty of a heart attack.

His father, also at age fifty, became blind from a degenerative disease of the retina. Later, his father suffered multiple strokes and died from hardening of the arteries at fifty-five years old.

His maternal grandmother was also afflicted by strokes and died at age sixty.

Many uncles and aunts added to his well-established family history of death by arterial occlusive disease.

Harold W. Harper, M.D. is quite aware that his background has him in perpetual danger — to be struck down anytime with acute symptoms of arteriosclerosis and to die in an instant.

When Dr. Harper was thirty-two years old and out of medical school just two years, his blood pressure stood at 220/150, and he weighed 358 pounds. Colleagues advised the new physician to leave the profession because the stress of medical practice was adding unduly to all his other atherosclerotic risk factors. Cardiologists offered him only two more years of survival.

By performing personal research on obesity and hypertension, Harold Harper developed a method that helped him lose 155 pounds. This massive weight loss somewhat decreased his high blood pressure, and thus reduced the danger from those two particular cardiac killers.

Being apprehensive of his irrevocable family history of arteriosclerosis, however, Dr. Harper took the precaution of carrying nitroglycerin tablets in his shaving kit wherever he traveled. He knew it was only a matter of time before he would be hit with a heart attack. His logic was that nitroglycerin might provide an immediate blood flow through the coronary arteries, until he could arrive at some emergency medical facility.

It came six years later, while he relaxed with friends aboard a sixty-five foot houseboat on Lake Powell, located between Arizona and Utah. They had been fishing and playing penny-ante poker.

Dr. Harper's first sensation of something gone wrong began with a headache "like little men inside my head with sledge hammers who were trying to get out," he later recalled. Another pain began just below his left breast at the rib margin. The pain rose slowly upward to his left shoulder, neck, jaw, and down the left arm. "This is it!" he told himself. "My time has come!"

In those first few seconds Dr. Harper felt as if a truck tire was weighing down upon his chest, with the truck still attached. It was a repressive feeling — a restrictive thing — which made him sweat profusely. Large beads of perspiration popped out on his forehead and ran like rivulets down his face. He rose to get the nitroglycerin from his shaving kit but, upon taking the first step, he fell flat on his face and broke his nose. There the man lay, face down, semi-conscious and unable to move or talk. His companions stared in shock at his still form. Although he attempted to manipulate an index finger to let his stunned friends know he was alive, even that the physician could not do.

The man who had been seated at Dr. Harper's left stood to help him, and he too fell like a sack of potatoes across the victim's body. The poker player on the right attempted to get up, but he collapsed across the table as well. The card player who sat opposite just slumped over.

The reason for these reactions was a not uncommon occurrence in boating. Their boat had been traveling at five knots in the face of a wind blowing exactly five knots. Gases coming from the motor had been held in place, stagnant. Internal combustion engines create carbon monoxide, which, when inhaled, combines with hemoglobin, the oxygen-carrying component of the blood. This limits the oxygen-supplying capability of the body and can be very dangerous. Among the first symptoms and signs are headache and unconsciousness. The four card players were poisoned by carbon monoxide engine exhaust, and carbon monoxide poisoning provoked Dr. Harper into a heart attack.

When he figured out the cause of his casualties' unconsciousness, the charter houseboat captain turned the boat into the wind, set the automatic pilot, and dragged the men onto the deck. Three of them finally were able to stand. The heart patient was awake but had no ability to move except to wiggle a few fingers. Dr. Harper was paralyzed. His friends let him lie on the deck breathing fresh air until their party arrived at a landing. By fast power-boat they took him to a small airport and flew him for hospitalization near his home.

By the time the fishermen reached Los Angeles, paralysis had left the patient and, at Dr. Harper's request, his friends took him to his office instead of to a hospital. There, using his own equipment, his medical staff gave the doctor an electrocardiogram, heart enzyme tests, and a full examination. The tests indicated that he was over the acute stage of the heart attack. He had undergone a limitation of circulatory exchange across the coronary vessels, the main point of his arterial weakness. Dr. Harper and the staff members decided that any hospitalization would be ineffective. He rested at home. The patient thereafter took time off from work for three days and then returned to medical practice on a modified work schedule which lasted for only three weeks. Then he worked full tilt as before.

Periodically the physician experienced anginal pain with pressure in the chest. His episodes of pain occurred when he worked very hard or walked up several flights of stairs without stopping to rest. He took no additional medical treatment, however, and kept at his regular routine that included twelve-hour work days.

"I continued with occasional chest pain for two years. I had been exploring for some way to get over the cardiac problem — do something for myself — but until then I knew that there was nothing to be done," Dr. Harper told me during the course of a few interviews. He knew that the usual medical treatments with vasodilators and low cholesterol or low fat diets were almost worthless. When doctors see the ineffectiveness of such a routine they naturally become skeptics. Since it is a leading cause of death, many physicians have come to regard arteriosclerotic heart disease as the normal attrition of old age. But that could not be the case for him. Dr. Harper was not quite ready to accept that old age philosophy for himself, since at that time he was just forty years old.

The Physician Learns of Chelation Therapy

"In February, 1972, I attended the annual meeting of the National Academy of Metabology in New York City. One of the lectures I tape recorded was delivered by H. Ray Evers, M.D. He spoke on the use of chelation therapy for heart disease. This doctor from a little town in Alabama had a dramatic story to tell about the treatment. Frankly, I didn't pay much attention. It just sounded too miraculous. I am, after all, a scientifically trained person unable to believe the type of miracle clinical response that Dr. Evers was describing," Dr. Harper admitted.

"Yet I couldn't push Evers' words out of my mind. That night in my hotel room I listened over again to the tape I had recorded. It made biochemical sense. I mulled it over for days. Back in Los Angeles I set a researcher to gathering all the literature about chelation that could be found. The medical librarians pulled out everything in their stacks and photocopied hundreds of pages of information.

"During his lecture, Dr. Evers had invited any physician who wanted to learn more about chelation to visit with him at the Columbia General Hospital in Andalusia, Alabama, where he then practiced. After delaying two weeks, my curiosity got the better of me. I had my secretary telephone to tell the man I was flying in to find out more — examine patient history charts — observe the people under care — and make a decision about his results."

"I reviewed 150 history charts and made hospital rounds with Dr. Evers beginning at 5:30 a.m. the next morning. He worked long hours. I noted patient response," said Dr. Harper. "People came from all over the U.S. — Florida, Alaska, Oregon, Wyoming, Connecticut, Maryland, Montana, and from foreign countries also. Patients had to be met at the plane because Andalusia is a tiny town 85 miles from the Montgomery (Alabama) Airport.

"People heard of the treatment through relatives. Word can get around fast when some unusually effective response is taking place," Dr. Harper continued. "I saw patients who had come with Raynaud's disease, others with purple extremities, gangrenous lesions on the legs and feet, and the whole range of arteriosclerotic conditions. And I saw these conditions heal. They healed well! I was shocked! I decided to go home and perform the technique on myself. Dr. Evers explained to me how I could acquire the chelating solution and make the mixture. I became my own first patient for chelation therapy.

"I took serial EKGs on myself during the treatment. After just three treatments my electrocardiograms returned to normal for the first time since I had entered medical school almost twelve years before. My EKGs have remained normal since. My blood pressure became normal. My anginal pain went away and has not returned. That has been for eight years now," Dr. Harper told me.

Chelation Therapy Helps to Widen Narrowed Arteries

The most promising treatment for premature aging of arteries, the most common form of which is atherosclerosis, is intravenous chelation therapy. This injection treatment apparently widens arteries that are narrowing and closing off blood flow. It reverses pathology of some of the most serious life-threatening problems that affect human beings, including coronary heart disease, stroke, peripheral vascular disease, gangrene of the extremities, high blood pressure, diabetes; kidney disorders of many types, including kidney stones; senility, reduced vision, thyroid and adrenal disturbances, psoriasis, scleroderma, emphysemia, Parkinson's disease, multiple sclerosis, hypercalcinosis, heavy metal poisoning, rheumatoid arthritis and some other forms of arthritis, and a variety of malfunctions and disabilities *where the basic issue is an interference with the flow of blood to a cell, tissue, organ or body part*.

Chelation therapy helps to deliver adequate nutrients and oxygen and removes toxic waste. The treatment acts through the mechanism of "chemical endarterectomy." It appears to be a sort of chemical "rotary-powered snake" that cleans out clogged blood vessels the way a septic engineer unclogs your home sewage pipes. Its action takes place at the microscopic or cellular level and there seems to be *no risk* of something breaking off and causing damage elsewhere.

The chelation technique makes use of a liquid "engineer," the chelation solution, which is a remarkable man-made amino acid called *ethylene diamine tetraacetic acid*, abbreviated EDTA. The EDTA solution has the unique property of binding with divalent or trivalent metals, including toxic heavy metals. It also combines with other minerals that when present in excess may bind with cellular constituents and apparently diminish the cellular enzyme function required to maintain cellular viability within the arteries. Thus the solution flushes the cells.

EDTA picks up ionic trace minerals complexed with various cell wall constituents and travels with them to the kidneys. There they are eliminated through the genitourinary tract. To a lesser extent the solution and combined constituents go through the liver and thence are sent out through the gastrointestinal tract. Testing reveals that a measurable and definite amount of ionized blood calcium is eliminated from the body this way. Almost none of this is the calcium that has been bound into bones and teeth, but rather it is metastatic or pathologic calcium lightly bound to components within the arterial wall and even to the walls of the platelets and blood cells. Thermograms taken before and after the chelation treatment reveal that areas of impaired circulation are frequently restored to normal by this fascinating and efficient liquid engineer called EDTA.

I have said that chelation heals a variety of malfunctions and disabilities where the basic issue is an interference in the blood supply. In fact, any system of treatment which brings fresh blood and oxygen to the tissues can be expected to aid in the healing process. Cleansing the blood by chelation does just that. When used properly, it is extremely scientific and highly effective.

When chelation is taken along with regular exercise, proper nutrition, and a balanced nutritional supplement program, the full-treatment regimen offers us the greatest promise for life extension and optimization of health. Early researchers have found chelation therapeutic benefits were "not lasting." The reason for that is clear now! No effort was made at that earlier time to improve the patients' lifestyles. No one enforced the full-treatment regimen then as knowledgeable chelation physicians require today. Unless a complete change in lifestyle is practiced, no medical therapy can succeed.

Chemical chelation cleans the blood of metastatic or pathological calcifications which are laid down on the intima, or from broken-off plaque which is floating free in the blood vessel lumen. *Metastatic calcium* is the stuff that combines with the proteins or the lipids in blood to help form atheromatous sclerosing plaques. *Metastatic calcium* impairs cellular function required to constantly repair damaged arteries. *Metastatic calcium* forms the hardening elements inside and around the walls of aging arteries. *Metastatic calcium* decreases circulation and interferes with life. Reverse the pathological calcification or prevent metastasis of calcium from happening in the first place, and we have markedly increased our chance to live our full life span.

The Natural Process of Chelation

The process of chelation is going on constantly in nature. It takes place in the bodies of living organisms, both plant and animal, as a natural function. Chelation is the means by which plants and animals are able to utilize inorganic minerals. For example, chlorophyll, the green matter of plants, is a chelate of magnesium. Hemoglobin, the oxygen-carrying pigment of human red blood cells, is a chelate of iron. The formation and function of enzymes, the protein substances which control most of our functions in the body, are all products of chelation. Aspirin, citric acid, and cortisone are known to function at least partially as chelating agents.

The chelation process, in fact, may be responsible for the effectiveness of almost all the drugs used in medicine to overcome disease. Without it they could not act and react with the body's physiology. Some of the most basic and yet complex chemical reactions found in nature and in man are encompassed by the chelation process.

As a process in plant and animal biology this reaction has been recognized for over thirty years. It is a biochemical process which is fundamental in:

- Food digestion and assimilation.
- The formation of numerous enzymes.
- The functions of enzyme systems.
- The synthesis of many hormones.
- The detoxifying of certain (toxic) chemicals.
- The detoxifying of certain metals, such as lead, arsenic, mercury, etc.
- The movement of vitamins, minerals, hormones and other nutrients across membranes of body tissues as part of transport systems.

The chelation mechanism controls many of our bodily functions. These same principles are applied in chelation therapy to treat hardening of the arteries and the diseases that result from this hardening effect.

The Definition of Chelation

The word *chelation* (pronounced *key-lay-shon*) is derived from the Greek word *chele* meaning *claw*, such as the claw of a lobster or crab. In effect, the chelate substance offers a firm, pincerlike binding of certain chemicals to a bivalent metal or other mineral. Chelation incorporates the metal or mineral ion into a heterocyclic ring structure. Certain chemicals are used to close this ring and grasp calcium or other metals with this claw-like action so that they are encircled or sequestered by the complex ring structure, thereby losing their toxic properties.

Writing in the September, 1962 *Illinois Medical Journal*, John H. Olwin, M.D., and J. L. Koppel, Ph.D., both from the Coagulation Research Laboratory, Department of Surgery, Presbyterian-St. Lukes' Hospital, Chicago, said:

> Chelation is the process by which certain chemical agents bind metals to form ring complexes. When such a chelate is formed, the cation becomes an integral

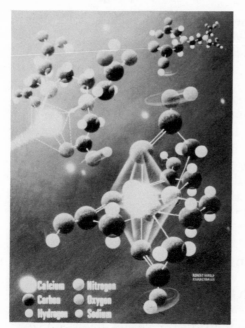

This illustration depicts how the molecule of ethylene diamine tetraacetic acid, or EDTA, works in the chelating process. The EDTA molecule, disodium salt, is shown in the upper right of the drawing, before chelation has begun. Then, in the upper left, the disodium EDTA attracts a divalent metal, calcium, the chief culprit for atherosclerotic plaque. The ionic calcium is drawn into the very center of the EDTA molecule. Finally, a chelate is created in the form of an octahedron (double pyramid), as the calcium ions are locked into an EDTA disodium salt ring. *(Drawing by Robert H. Knabenbauer, supplied courtesy of World Life Research Institute.)*

part of a stable ring structure and ceases to act as a free ion. The stabilities of the resulting chelates depend upon the cation involved, one which is more weakly bound being displaced by another which is more strongly bound. It is upon this property that the clinical usefulness of chelation therapy depends.

The disodium salt of ethylene diamine tetra acetate, or EDTA, is the weakly bound cation replaced by other cation minerals higher up in the electromotive scale. A *cation* is an ion carrying a charge of positive electricity. Thus, disodium EDTA forms stronger soluble complexes with cations such as barium, beryllium, cadmium, calcium, chromium, cobalt, copper, lead, iron, magnesium, manganese, mercury, nickel, strontium and zinc. That's why, as Drs. Olwin and Koppel suggest:

> The use of chelating agents in the treatment of certain clinical conditions is not new. It is perhaps best known for its benefits in heavy metal, particularly lead, poisoning. Its use in other conditions, such as scleroderma, porphyria, cardiac arrhythmias, and atherosclerosis in some of its clinical manifestations, is less well known.

EDTA grasps metals, including calcium, with this claw-like action and encircles or sequesters them within a complex ring. They lose their physiologic and toxic properties this way. Therefore, when chelation takes place, the calcium or heavy metal comes in contact with EDTA, or some other chelating agent, and becomes imprisoned by the ring. The sodium is never dropped and so the sodium is apparently not toxic. It is simply excreted by the body intact with the EDTA. Excess lead or other toxic metals are excreted from the system along with the EDTA. The "toxic" element is trapped by the chelator, like the claw of a crab holding something in its pincers.

The ability of EDTA amino acid to grasp or bind with the ionic calcium found in metastatic or pathological calcium deposits is phenomonal. It seems to be catalytic in its power to excrete or mobilize calcium far beyond the dose of the medicine itself. Some of this reaction takes place because of the parathormone (the hormone of the parathyroid gland) response to the induced hypocalcemia during the infusion of the drug. I will describe in depth the mechanism of action of EDTA in Chapters Four and Five.

As potential users of this life-extending treatment, we should be aware that chelation is as old as life on this planet. All biological processes are involved in the phenomenon. It is only in recent years, however, that chelation has emerged as a very valuable therapeutic technique for purposes of predictable health improvement.

The History of EDTA Chelation

In interviews with Bruce W. Halstead, M.D., who is a biotoxicologist and Director of the World Life Research Institute in Colton, California, I learned that EDTA was first synthesized by Mr. F. Munz, a German chemist. Then it was developed by the I. G. Farben Industries as a result of the geopolitical problems created by Adolf Hitler. Germany required the product in its fabrics and textiles industries. In due course, EDTA was patented in 1930, as reported in the *American Journal of Laboratory and Clinical Medicine* ("Regarding EDTA," 1930). Working with some older components, I. G. Farben finally brought out the agent in 1931 as a substitute for citric acid as a coating or preservative of fibers.

Chelation therapy was first employed in medicine in 1941 with the use of sodium citrate in lead poisoning. This usage was reported in an article, "Treatment of lead poisoning with sodium citrate" by S. S. Kety and T. V. Letonoff (*Proc. Soc. Exp. Biol. MED. 46* (1941), 476-477).

EDTA was patented in the United States in 1949 by Frederick Bersworth, a biochemist at Georgetown University, for the Martin-Dennis Company. Several papers on EDTA were published in the early 1950s.

Dr. Halstead said, "EDTA is known to all analytical chemists. There are entire books devoted to it. The number of articles in the field of analytical chemistry dealing with EDTA number into the thousands. One of the values of this agent is its precise nature. At least in an *in vitro* situation (in the test tube) you can literally mathematically predict how EDTA is going to act and approximately to what extent it is going to chelate."

In a March, 1976 appearance before the Advisory Panel on Internal Medicine of the Scientific Board of the California Medical Association (CMA), which I shall describe in detail in Chapter Eleven, Norman E. Clarke, Sr., M.D., a cardiologist of Birmingham, Michigan, told the Scientific Board of his pioneering activities with chelation therapy.

"I learned about EDTA in 1953 from Dr. Albert J. Boyle, Professor of Chemistry at Wayne State University, Detroit, and from Dr. Gordon B. Myers, who then was Professor of Medicine at the same university and a well-known cardiologist. Drs. Boyle and Myers had preliminary experience in treating two patients at University Hospital, Detroit who had calcified mitral (heart) valves. The patients were almost completely incapacitated," Dr. Clarke told the CMA. "The doctors were pleased with the results (of chelation treatment) because they obtained very satisfactory return of cardiac function. But they [Drs. Boyle and Myers] did not have the opportunity or the time to go on with it (their research). Dr. Boyle asked if I would — because then I was chairman of the research department of Providence Hospital, Detroit — undertake a study of EDTA in cardiovascular diseases, which I did.

"I knew, having been in cardiology quite a number of years [since 1921], that arteriosclerotic cardiovascular disease was a helpless, hopeless situation for the cardiologist. I had to start by trying to find out whether it was safe [EDTA]; what was the best dosage; were there any side effects; and how would we standardize its use as a treatment?

"Well, of course," Dr. Clarke continued, "the first couple of years we treated only hospital patients where we had them under excellent control. We started with rather large dosage [10 gm.] and had some side reactions consisting primarily of signs of a B-6 [Vitamin B-6—pyridoxine] deficiency. Some males' scrotum lost a complete cast of skin, but it was absolutely painless and with no sensation of discomfort. After finding the proper dosage, of course, all those things have never happened again. And even with those large doses we had no unusual or serious side effects. Ultimately we determined, and for a long time gave, five grams, and later determined that three grams was the proper dose.

"In the last twenty-three years of my experience with EDTA chelation I would say conservatively, because after all those years you don't keep accurate records with all you do, but conservatively I have given at least 100,000 to 120,000 infusions of EDTA and seen nobody harmed," the chelation specialist said. "I've never seen any serious toxicity whatsoever. I've seen only benefits . . . ."

The veteran cardiologist went on to describe more success with diabetes and other cases of rest pain. Then Dr. Clarke said, "Another field in which I have found [EDTA] most effective is cerebrovascular senility. I am extremely impressed with that, not only by the improvement in the patients but from the economic factor today. All you have to do is go into one of those old folks' homes and see the senile people sitting around and you'll recognize immediately not only the economic problems but the physical and mental problems that they and their families go through."

Dr. Clarke, who is eighty-eight years old himself, concluded his remarks to the California Medical Association's advisory panel assembled to hear about chelation therapy. He said, "After all these years and with all that experience, I am just as certain as can be that EDTA chelation therapy is the best treatment that has ever been brought out for occlusive vascular disease."

With Dr. Clarke's longtime successful experience with EDTA, it is almost appalling that the medical profession in the U.S. has continued to reject it.

Chapter Three

The Therapeutic Effects
EDTA Chelation Achieves

As the chemical EDTA floats past a hardened area in a blood vessel wall, its strong attraction for calcium will literally zap the calcium right out of the hardened area which is like taking the rivets out of a bridge structure. If you take out enough rivets, the bridge will collapse. And this is what happens to the hardened area. After enough calcium is removed from it, it collapses and is reabsorbed by the body. The calcium which has been kidnapped by the amino acid is excreted through the kidneys into the urine and removed from the body. The net result is more room for the blood to flow through the vessel and a better circulation.

— H. Rudolph Alsleben, M.D.,
*How to Survive the New Health
Catastrophes*, 1973

Chelation Therapy Alters the Course of Parkinson's Disease

In a hotel room in Kansas City, Missouri during the September 1976 semi-annual meeting of the American Academy of Medical Preventics, I was able to gather together nine physicians to discuss their experiences with administering chelation therapy. One of them was Sibyl W. Anderson, D.O., who practices osteopathic medicine with her husband, Leon Anderson, D.O., in Jenks, Oklahoma. This is what Sibyl Anderson told me:

"My husband, Dr. Leon Anderson, was the first patient we ever treated with chelation, six years ago. He had a tremor in his right hand and experienced difficulty performing routine functions such as tying his shoelaces. He went for an examination to our favorite neurologist in Tulsa, Oklahoma. The doctor was unable to give a definite diagnosis of Parkinson's disease, *paralysis agitans*, because it was in such an early stage, but he couldn't say he didn't have Parkinsonism. He did not offer any treatment or advice except that Dr. Leon should come back if it got worse."

Parkinson's disease, also known as *shaking palsy*, is a neurological syndrome usually resulting from arteriosclerotic changes in the basal ganglia. It is characterized by rhythmical muscular tremors, rigidity of movement, a peculiar rapid or hastening acceleration of gait, droopy posture, and masklike countenance of the patient.

"Whether the problem was in the hand or the brain, we felt the best thing we could do was to get good nutrition to the tissues so the body could do its own healing," Dr. Sibyl said. "We worked on my husband's dietary and vitamin and mineral supplement program, but the fundamental key to curative treatment that we used was EDTA chelation.

"After only five EDTA treatments Dr. Leon really began to see a difference in his tremor. He could use his hand for all the little things we have to do for ourselves that you don't actually think about until you can't do them. He took thirty chelation treatments altogether and has never had a problem with Parkinson-like symptoms since that time. Dr. Leon has taken a short series of intravenous EDTA yearly," Dr. Sibyl Anderson said.

EDTA Chelation Reverses Blindness

She described another person, a prominent, fifty-eight-year-old attorney from Tulsa, Oklahoma, who visited Drs. Sibyl and Leon Anderson in October 1972. The man asked if they could help him get better nutrition to his retina. He had been blind in one eye for seven years. One month prior to his visit to the two osteopathic physicians he had lost the central vision of his other eye.

The patient already had made the rounds of the best eye specialists in Tulsa, Oklahoma City, and San Francisco. After going through thorough evaluations and laser beam treatments, he had been sent home with no hope of ever being able to see to read, except with aid from an inverted television camera. The attorney was told by the ophthalmologists that he could never again drive a car or perform many of the essential activities necessary for a busy law practice. The patient's diagnosis of *macular degeneration* was made by each of his three ophthalmologists.

The *macula retinae* is a small, orange-yellow oval area, three by five millimeters, on the inner surface of the retina slightly below the optic disk near the rear pole of the eyeball, and therefore is the visual axis. At its center is the *fovea centralis*, which provides the best visual acuity under photopic conditions. If it degenerates, as in macular degeneration, blindness results. This is what happened to the Tulsa attorney.

The attorney's wife had read Adelle Davis' book, *Let's Get Well*. Adelle Davis had mentioned that the use of vitamin A injections and other nutrients were helpful with treatment of *retinitis pigmentosa*, another retina problem. The couple wondered if injections of vitamin A might be useful as an aide for the near-blind patient in his particular problem as well. They thought it might be worth a try.

"Dr. Leon and I discussed nutrition in general with the couple, gave specific diet instructions, and prescribed an oral vitamin program. Also we injected both vitamin A and vitamin E," Dr. Sibyl Anderson said. "Even with this approach we needed to get the nutrients to the retina directly, so our first thought was chelation treatments which we felt would open up the retinal blood supply.

"Since we had not treated a patient with macular degeneration before, we called Dr. H. Rudolph Alsleben in Anaheim, California, whom we had heard was treating a number of patients daily with intravenous chelation," said Dr. Sibyl. "Dr. Alsleben encouraged us to start treatments immediately. He said that he had some very good response with retinal problems.

"Our own patient's vision at this time was 20/400 (legally blind) in the right eye, and he had no corrective lens on the left eye, having lost the central vision in that eye seven years previously," the osteopathic physician told me.

"The attorney's wife was very conscientious in following the nutritional program and giving her husband his supplements. Her cooperation was essential in his treatment. They were both very disciplined and delightful to work with," she said. "We proceeded to administer chelation therapy."

I asked Dr. Anderson about her patient's progress as a result of the treatment.

She said, "At the end of two and one-half months he was able to read the newspaper with a special corrective lens, and at three and one-half months he could resume driving and read normally with the new corrective lens. Also at this time, the left eye had improved sufficiently for a corrective lens. It is interesting to note that the medical literature states that a patient with macular degeneration can expect continual loss of vision and should change his occupation and mode of living to adjust to his problem."

By his taking intravenous EDTA chelation, no change of occupation was needed for this patient. The attorney, I am told by other physicians who know the case, is highly successful in the practice of law in Tulsa today. He is exceedingly well known in that city.

Dr. Anderson concluded, "Over a year's time this attorney took 105 treatments. During this period several doctors contributed their expertise, including Dr. H. Ray Evers and Dr. Morgan Raiford. My patient's visual acuity at the end of one year was 20/35. He continues to take the intravenous EDTA treatments periodically."

By January 6, 1977, when last I checked with Dr. Sibyl Anderson, the attorney had taken a total of 134 chelations. "His general health also has *much* improved," she said.

Intravenous Chelation Aids Multiple Sclerosis

While researching this book in another part of the country in December 1976, I learned of a man living in the vicinity of my home who had taken intravenous chelation to aid multiple sclerosis. I was told that he had walked with the assistance of two canes when he arrived at the chelation clinic. After receiving just one week of chelation treatment he gave up the use of one cane and walked with better balance and more strength. Prior to that, he had been under ordinary medical care for multiple sclerosis and his condition had not shown any improvement. This man had not been made aware that he was an MS patient until May, 1973, although his family knew possibly a year before that.

Back at my desk about a month later, I followed this lead and interviewed Alvin Kavaler, fifty years old, of West Hartford, Connecticut. Mr. Kavaler is a former insurance salesman who is confined to his home presently because of his MS condition. He confirmed some of the things I had heard about his improvement following chelation therapy, but not all of them.

Mr. Kavaler said, "I would be reluctant to say that chelation therapy is any kind of cure for multiple sclerosis. It's not! Although I experienced improvement after taking the treatment, I think probably it came from a change in some other physical problems I had that I didn't know about. In any case, I have encouraged many MS affected people to go for chelation since the treatment is an aid to relieving symptoms of poor circulation. I am convinced that most of our discomforts as MS patients come from circulatory difficulties. Unfortunately, the usual M.D. seems to think that anything bothering an MS victim is due to MS. Not so! For instance, my feet had always felt ice cold. This condition had been bothersome for as long as I can remember. A few weeks after I took my first eighteen bottles of chelation solution I realized that my feet — and the rest of me, too — were warm, and they have remained warm. This comfort has been an exciting new experience for me — to have a warm-feeling body, hands and feet all of the time. I know that many multiple sclerosis patients are troubled by feelings of coldness all over."

Multiple sclerosis is a chronic, slowly progressive disease of the central nervous system characterized clinically by a lot of symptoms and signs which come and go intermittently. There are visual disturbances, transient weakness, stiffness or fatigability of a limb, interference with walking, bladder control difficulties, occasional dizziness, and other troubles that slowly get worse.

Obviously, chelation is no cure-all, but the attitude of American medicine is too often do nothing except for what is accepted by the medical mainstream.

A Chelation Pioneer Tells of Giving 16,000 Infusions

John H. Olwin, M.D., Clinical Professor of Surgery at Rush Medical College in Chicago, a seventy-year-old vascular surgeon whose co-authored paper I quoted from in Chapter Two, described his experiences with giving chelation therapy. Dr. Olwin made an appearance before the ad hoc committee of the Advisory Panel on Internal Medicine of the Scientific Board of the California Medical Association. His appearance occurred immediately before Dr. Clarke made his presentation, which I described in the last chapter. From the notarized transcript of that hearing, and with the permission of Garry F. Gordon, M.D. of Sacramento, California, who is the immediate past President of the American Academy of Medical Preventics, and Yiwen

Y. Tang, M.D., F.A.B.F.P. of San Francisco, who had requested the hearing, I offer Dr. Olwin's testimony about the therapeutic effects that EDTA chelation achieves.

First Dr. Olwin recounted how he became acquainted with EDTA chelation. "Some sixteen years ago," he said, "a biochemist in the department of surgery of one of our medical schools asked me if I were using chelation therapy on my patients with obliterative atherosclerosis. I asked him what chelation therapy was, and he explained. I subsequently talked with Dr. Clarke, Dr. Al Boyle, and Drs. Lawrence E. Meltzer and J. Roderick Kitchell, who are co-authors of papers on chelation, and who practice in Philadelphia.

"I then went to the Veteran's Hospital in Hines, Illinois where I was the attending [physician] on the vascular service," Dr. Olwin said. "There I began using this treatment according to the schedule of Drs. Kitchell and Meltzer on our patients on whom we had written off the legs because of obliterative atherosclerosis. We were awaiting these patients' consent for amputation. We began using this material [EDTA] and saved a number of limbs. The necrotic dead areas of skin or flesh were limited; they dropped off; the limbs warmed; the nails and hair began to grow [following administration of chelation therapy], and after several of these experiences I began to use EDTA chelation in my private practice.

"Over the past fifteen years," Dr. Olwin told the CMA review committee members, "I have used it for between 335 and 350 patients, representing something over 16,000 infusions of about three grams each, in most instances. Seventy-five of these patients have been on chelation therapy for more than five years, and twenty-five of those seventy-five for more than ten years."

Dr. Olwin asked and answered a compelling question: "What are the effects that we observe? Well first there is relief of claudication. Patients can walk farther. Some of them say they can walk as far as they could normally.

"There is relief of the ischemic pain.

"There is a warming of the limbs, both subjective and objective.

"There is an arrest of gangrene.

"There is a regrowth of hair and nails.

"There is a relief of angina.

"There is healing of the ischemic ulcers . . .

"Some patients with thrombophlebitis migrans, even those on controlled anticoagulant therapy, will have recurring episodes of thromboembolism, but we are able to reduce this materially—in some instances eliminate the recurrence of thrombophlebitis—by adding to the anticoagulant routine intermittent doses of EDTA," the vascular surgeon said. (*Thrombophlebitis migrans* is a creeping or slowly advancing inflammation of a vein with secondary thrombus formation. It appears in first one vein and then another.)

"Another observed effect is the increase in capillary blood flow. You can observe the flow in the conjunctival [eye membrane] vessels. There is extreme sludging of blood in most patients with atherosclerosis. Without exception, over a period of time, the flow in capillaries as seen in the eye is improved after treatment of several months with EDTA.

"We have seen improvement in mental processes," Dr. Olwin assured his reviewing peers. "In the early stages we noted that these people with gangrenous limbs and gangrenous toes were not as mentally sharp as they had once been. One young executive who had lost his job because of mental disturbances returned to work after he had been treated with EDTA.

"Some of our neurologists became interested in this and with their cooperation, we treated thirteen patients with chronic brain syndrome. Four of these [patients] showed clinical improvement. Three of them showed reversal of [abnormal] EEGs [electroencephalograms] and one of them had a return to a normal EEG, a man in his late seventies. He went on to die at the age of eighty-three of a perforated duodenal ulcer.

"We see an improvement in ECGs [another way to abbreviate EKG electrocardiograms]. This is not my field, but some of my colleagues have observed and some of my patients have experienced an improvement in this [heart] condition."

Psychological and Internal Medical Benefits As Well

Dr. Olwin, a peripheral vascular specialist, ordinarily works fifteen hours a day operating on blood vessels and amputating limbs. Yet here is a vascular surgeon who dramatically saves arms and legs by the intravenous infusion of a chemical. Where possible, he substitutes medicine for surgery.

He said, "I've been taking this chelation for myself for ten years, almost every third week for maybe five years, and now about every two weeks. As far as I know, my chemistry's normal. All my functions are normal. And I expect to continue to work for an indefinite period."

There were a number of psychological and internal medical benefits that Dr. Olwin observed in addition to his work with peripheral vascular disease. For instance, it was reported by some of his patients that they enjoyed an increase in libidinous drive and sexual potency. He told the California Medical Association reviewers the following anecdote:

"An eighty-year-old brilliant lawyer in Chicago had had a chronic brain syndrome for many years. His neurologist asked about this chelation treatment; I explained the experience that we'd had, and the family wished to have the elderly man treated. The patient was treated in collaboration with the neurologist, and after about a year there was no improvement in his [the patient's] chronic brain syndrome.

"However, the eighty-year-old man's wife called me one day and asked, 'Is this supposed to increase sexual desire?' I said, 'We've had that recorded.' And she replied, 'Well, James has not been interested in sex for fifteen years and last night he tried to make love to me!'

"Perhaps this effect was an indication that the man's sexual problem was not a functional affair but an organic change. It seems reasonable that if blood supply is being improved, all organs of the body may benefit from this improvement," Dr. Olwin conjectured.

In other instances the specialist cited the reduction of insulin requirement for diabetics. He said, "One of our patients, a juvenile diabetic, who was almost blind and taking seventy-five units of insulin, had, after a series of treatments, a reduction to thirty-five units of insulin."

The vascular surgeon showed color slides during his CMA presentation. The slides included indisputable tables of results and "before and after" photographs of patients with a variety of problems. His tables and charts indicated blood fat metabolism alterations.

Dr. Olwin said, "We observed a reduction in lipid levels in all patients in which we have done any studies on lipid levels. This [chelation effect] must be an enzymatic action. The mechanism is still unclear. The lipid reduction returns to the pretherapy levels after four to six weeks on termination of the therapy. And [lipid levels] can again be reduced after the therapy is restarted. In three instances we have had recanalization of main arterial channels."

(To explain: Dr. Olwin said that he saw a *recanalization*, a new opening, in major blood vessels after there had previously been complete blockage in these vessels by thrombotic occlusion. The new arterial opening forms by organization of the thrombus with creation by the body of new capillaries that let blood flow through, where before, blockage prevented it. That is *collateral circulation* or recanalization. The body part that is about to die of blood starvation now will receive blood nutrition and live.)

Dr. Olwin added, "I had one patient, a man who had claudication for six months; after about twenty-two months [of chelation], his pulses recurred in his feet and arteriography clearly indicated that there had been a recanalization of an obstruction at the level of the abductor tendon [in the lower thighs]." (The patient Dr. Olwin was telling about, a war veteran, had actually been rolled on a stretcher bed into the operating room to have his leg amputated. But Dr. Olwin put in an arterial graft as a bypass instead and immediately started him on chelation therapy.) "The graft closed several weeks later, but there had apparently been enough of the effect of EDTA that his gangrene sloughed. And this is the foot at some weeks later." The slide that Dr. Olwin flashed on the screen showed the man's foot was healed—his leg saved.

He described another patient: "A woman of forty-five had had endarterectomy [surgical removal of an artery's lining along with its occluding atheromatous deposits] of both common iliac arteries [major blood vessels in the abdominal area that supply the entire lower portion of the body]. About three months later, despite anti-coagulant therapy, these arteries closed,"

Dr. Olwin said. "Chelation was started; anticoagulants were continued; around eighteen months later she reopened both iliac arteries. These arteries have remained open under continuous anticoagulants and intermittent chelation therapy," Dr. Olwin told the CMA investigating panel.

Chelation Therapy Improves Memory

During our many interviews, Warren M. Levin, M.D., F.A.A.F.P. of New York City, described his personal experience with giving himself chelation therapy. He said, "I went through a full preventive medical checkup including cardiac stress testing and was pronounced 'fit as a fiddle.' However, my father had died at the age of fifty-six with a coronary. Also, I'm short, relatively stocky, and have been eating what I now consider unhealthy food for the first forty years of my life—until I learned better. I know that I have been undergoing the same sort of degenerative changes of hardening of the arteries like everyone else. I think that in the past few years, by altering my lifestyle with regular daily exercise and better eating habits, I have slowed down the pathology. Nevertheless, I wanted to do more than just slow it down. I wanted to eliminate atherosclerosis from my body altogether, if I could. So despite my feeling in really fine health, I took a series of twenty chelation treatments in the spring of 1975.

"About eight weeks after I finished self-administered chelation, I suddenly realized that a very important memory change had taken place in me. My memory was much improved," said Dr. Levin. "I have always been blessed with a pretty good brain — high I.Q. and all that — and now I am able to remember long unused addresses and telephone numbers. I had no problem with that kind of remembering. My annoyances would occur in the middle of a workday in this unbelievably hectic office — allergy tests being taken — chelations being given to patients — physical examinations going on — and other activities.

"I might be examining one person and have another waiting in my consulation room," Dr. Levin continued. "The telephones would be ringing. My nurse might ask me about service charges or appointments for patients — sixteen different inputs coming at me at once. Then I may walk into my consultation room from the examining room and have to stop to ask myself, 'What did I come in here for?' Often I'd have to turn around and go back to the examining room to see my patient or look at the chart, and then it would come to me. I'd realize, 'Oh yes, I was supposed to get that order blank' or fill out the form on my desk."

Dr. Levin assured me, "That sort of memory lapse doesn't happen to me anymore. The whole pattern has modified dramatically. There is absolutely no question in my mind that my improved memory is a direct result of chelation therapy. I took a few more treatments in 1976 and 1977, and I will be taking chelation at fairly regular intervals indefinitely. It's the best *preventative medicine* that we have to offer in this country to eliminate hardening of the arteries for somebody in my state of health and at my age of forty-five years."

Other Benefits of EDTA Chelation

What? A treatment to improve the memory, stop parkinsonism, aid multiple sclerosis, reverse blindness, recanalize blocked arterial channels, lower insulin requirements for diabetics, restore libido and sexual potency, dissolve thromboses, reverse gangrene, relieve claudication pain — EDTA chelation does all that? Yes, this is the conclusion I have come to after much investigation. The medical scientists and many patients whom I talked with assure me those are the facts. And there is more.

In their book, *How to Survive the New Health Catastrophes,* H. Rudolph Alsleben, M.D. and Wilfrid E. Shute, M.D. explain some additional chelation therapeutic effects that occur with intravenous administration of the synthesized amino acid, disodium ethylene diamine tetraacetic acid (EDTA). This substance provides the following beneficial effects:[1] It —
- prevents the deposit of cholesterol in the liver.
- reduces blood cholesterol levels.
- causes high blood pressure to drop in 60 percent of the cases.
- reverses the toxic effects of digitalis excess.
- converts to normal 50 percent of cardiac arrhythmias.
- reduces or relaxes excessive heart contractions.
- increases intracellular potassium.
- reduces heart irritability.
- increases the removal of lead.
- removes calcium from atherosclerotic plaques.
- dissolves kidney stones.
- reduces serum iron and protects against iron poisoning and iron storage disease.
- reduces heart valve calcification and improves heart function.
- detoxifies several poisonous venoms.
- reduces the dark pigmentation of varicose veins.
- heals calcified necrotic ulcers.
- reduces the disabling effects of intermittent claudication.
- improves vision in diabetic retinopathy.
- decreases macular degeneration.
- dissolves small cataracts.

Review of the medical literature on this subject indicates that the value of EDTA chelation therapy has been well tested and carefully reported. Some major institutions have underwritten studies of the intravenous therapy. Grants-in-aid for research on EDTA chelation therapy have been given by:
1. The National Institutes of Health
2. The U.S. Public Health Service
3. The National Institute of Arthritis and Metabolic Diseases

4. The University of California, Los Alamos Scientific Laboratory
5. The American Cancer Society
6. The Charles S. Hayden Foundation
7. The Elsa U. Pardee Foundation
8. The Oscar Meyer Foundation
9. The U.S. Atomic Energy Commission
10. The John A. Hartford Foundation
11. The Providence Hospital Research Department, Detroit, Michigan
12. The Equitable Life Assurance Society, Bureau of Medical Research
13. The U.S. Public Health Department, Division of General Medical Sciences
14. The Mayo Clinic and Mayo Foundation

The scientific literature search I conducted in 1976 and 1977 in order to write this book, and a 1974 review carried out by Paul H. Huff, Ph.D. of Fullerton, California both indicate that there has been a high degree of success in achievement of therapeutic benefits through the use of chelation therapy.

Just what does EDTA chelation therapy do inside the body? What is the substance's mechanism of action? How is it able to unharden arteries, widen arterial tunnels, and make so many people feel a variety of benefits? The next chapter will answer these questions. But already I believe my research has shown this to be a possible viable treatment for many ailments connected with hardening of the arteries.

Chapter Four

The Internal Mechanism of EDTA Chelation

Preventive medicine has moved into the space age, where the latest technology is employed to detect the earliest deterioration, so that maximum extension of useful life span may be attained. . . . Since chelation therapy appears to offer a nontoxic life extension in research animals and beneficial effects in man, it is clearly desirable to increase its efficacy. To do this most efficiently, all possible mechanisms of action should be identified.

— Garry F. Gordon, M.D.
and Robert B. Vance, D.O.,
Osteopathic Annals, February, 1976

Nick Jurich Wins the War Waging in His Arteries

Our arteries are ongoing battle scenes. They fight skirmishes with the pernicious forces in our unhealthy environment. All of us undergo the same sort of internal strife, and most of us succumb eventually to effects of this pathogenic stress. Our arteries develop atheromatous plaques that choke off our blood supply to the limbs, the heart, or the brain.

Crippling deformity and finally death almost came to Nicholas Jurich, a real estate broker in Pittsburgh, Pennsylvania. In 1971 Mr. Jurich had a serious brush with the pathogenic stress common in our industrialized environment. It took the form of a rear-end automobile collision. The resulting whiplash injury he suffered set off a chain reaction of severe physical complications.

During the two years that followed his accident, Nick Jurich's metabolism went awry. He was afflicted with a near-fatal trace mineral deficiency, malfunctioning of his glandular organs, aggravation of a dormant arthritic condition, and intense chest pains. Most alarming were the spells of unconsciousness that struck him without warning from an unknown cause. Repeated bouts of sudden blackouts landed the man in the hospital.

The Pittsburgh physicians put the patient through numerous laboratory tests that turned up no specific diagnosis. The doctors confessed they were puzzled and called in consultants. In futility, the several specialists finally prescribed Dilantin to be taken by Jurich for at least one year and possibly for the rest of his life. The use of such a medication was an outright experiment, since nothing but symptoms were being treated. They failed to find the source of the patient's problem and prescribed empirically. But harsh toxic effects from Dilantin, such as slurred speech, constant drowsiness, blurred vision, and continuous tiredness could have ensued if Nick Jurich had followed the physicians' orders. He did not!

An enthusiastic referral by a visiting friend, who owned a health food store, motivated Nick Jurich to telephone from his Pittsburgh hospital room for an appointment with Dr. Ray Evers. The patient left his bed and flew south for diagnosis and eventual treatment.

Jurich received a total of 117 blood vessel-flushing chelations, administered intermittently from June 16, 1973 to November 30, 1975.

"My various symptoms cleared up," Jurich told me. The blackouts disappeared. They had come from a severe deficiency of body minerals and inadequate oxygen supplied to the brain by his inadequate arterial circulation. The chelation treatments restored the circulation by opening formerly blocked blood vessels. "Where I walked with great difficulty before from a prior acute onset of rheumatoid arthritis, now I could walk longer distances, although a little awkwardly. My joint swelling went down and most of the pain went away. My metabolism stablized, glandular functioning seemed to improve considerably; my energy and mental alertness returned. Dr. Evers not only used chelation therapy, but he also built me up with an optimum diet, vitamins and chelated minerals. Now I'm able to hike far and wide without feeling any claudication pain in my legs," the man said.

Jurich spoke with enthusiasm to friends about his treatment results, so that others with symptoms of hardening of the arteries also made the trip to Dr. Evers' clinic. "In our community we've seen case after case of wonderful recovery from a variety of circulatory conditions," he said. "Carmen Carulli, a Braddock, Pennsylvania policeman is one of them. Carmen read an article about my friends who had chelation in the *Pittsburgh Press* of February 8, 1975. During that week he was waiting for Texas heart surgeon Dr. Denton Cooley to accept him for an examination appointment.

"Carmen traveled south for chelation care instead of going through open heart surgery. He took almost seven weeks of chelation treatment. Believe it or not, now Carmen Carulli is back at work without the need of any heart operation," Jurich said.

The Story Police Officer Carmen Carulli Told

I searched for Officer Carulli to check out his story. This is what he told me:

"In September, 1969 I had a severe heart attack and was put in intensive care for three weeks. I was out of work for three months and then returned to the force.

"Three years later I again began to get this awful angina pain and finally needed hospitalization. This time I returned to work within a few weeks.

"About a year and a half later, one night while on duty at two o'clock in the morning, I picked up a man off the street and was socked for a third time by terrible chest pains — the same angina as before. The doctors quickly put me in the hospital. I was hospitalized that time for four weeks, and a heart specialist from Pittsburgh performed an angiogram on me. That angiogram caused me awful angina pain while I laid there on the table. When the catheter went in and hit an artery I felt terrible, and the doctors quickly pulled it out. The angiogram showed that I had three coronary artery blockages, 85 percent clogging of one, 80 percent in another, and 75 percent in the third.

"My cardiologist said that I was beyond surgery — that I was a goner! Well, I couldn't accept such a depressing outlook, so after some time I called down to Houston, Texas to make an appointment for an evaluation by Dr. Denton Cooley. His secretary scheduled me for an examination in a week. But six days later, as I was getting ready to catch a plane for Houston, the same secretary phoned to say that Dr. Cooley couldn't see me because he was attending a convention, or something. It looked to me like I might die and nobody would care. That's when I found out about Dr. Evers and chelation therapy," Carmen Carulli told me.

"I telephoned Dr. Evers and made an appointment to see him. Even though I was confined to a wheelchair — I was that weak — had angina at any exertion — my friends made sure that I managed the trip. One or the other of them pushed my wheelchair on and off the plane. I brought along my bag full of medicines. There were all kinds of heart pills that I thought I could not live without.

"After he examined me, Dr. Evers had me throw all the darn pills in the garbage, and he started the chelation injections. When I took three bottles of that EDTA stuff I started walking around the hospital. The fourth day I walked three city blocks, and each day I added on distance.

"Remember what I'm telling you! When I went down there I was in a wheelchair — couldn't walk at all because of the angina pain," emphasized the policeman. "At the sixth day about fifteen of us, all were Dr. Evers' patients, went to New Orleans to see the city. It was a windy, blustery day. I walked fifteen blocks in that gusty wind without any recurrence of my chest pain. And I haven't had any angina since. I stayed in Dr. Evers' hospital for six-and-a-half weeks and returned to get ready for work one week after I came home. Then I went back to work.

"The Braddock Police Department wouldn't let me come back on duty unless I did my job. I put in a full eight hours daily walking the beat, and police work is pretty rough nowadays. I get into some scraps — bodily pick up 200-pound drunks off the street — walk up apartment house steps maybe three, four, five flights at a time. I'm obligated to do whatever I'm assigned, and I do it. I wouldn't be around here if it wasn't for the grace of God, Dr.

Evers and chelation therapy," said police officer Carmen Carulli.

Officer Carulli is robust, wide-shouldered, vigorous, built like a bull, and as tough a cop as you would see on any ghetto street corner in New York, Chicago or Detroit. He spoke emphatically and demanded pre-publication approval of what I would write about him. Carulli did not change anything when I sent him copy for correcting in February 1977, except that he gave *God* part of the credit for his recovery. And Nick Jurich told me many more impressive stories of arterial occlusion being reversed.

By now, you may be wondering about the mechanism by which this widening of narrowed arteries takes place. I will present a full disclosure of the internal decalcification process using EDTA chelation therapy in the balance of this chapter and in the next.

Information Sources Advising Me on the Chelation Mechanism

Recognizing that until now therapies available for patients suffering with arteriosclerosis have truly been inadequate, the physician who is conscientious and who reads the information to follow will not disdain its value. Chelation therapy deserves study. The material is frankly awesome when one considers that its use can save a million or more lives each year, lives ordinarily lost to hardening of the arteries.

I am going to popularize some highly technical medical information in order to educate you, my nonmedical reader. I shall try to avoid teaching any kind of medical school course in human vascular physiology. However, it will be necessary for doctor and patient to have all the facts.

The well-informed physician, before administering this treatment, will want to review the entire literature on cardiovascular chemotherapy that employs synthetic chelating agents. The chief agent among them is *disodium edetate*, known generically as *disodium ethylene diamine tetra-acetic acid (EDTA)*. For that reason, although I don't anticipate the lay reader will make use of all the scientific references that supplement my information, many such references are included in the footnotes, primarily for the doctor's benefit.

It is possible that this book may be the first place a physician comes across a full description of the chelation therapeutic technique. The victim of hardening of the arteries or a victim's family member may bring this book to the physician to ask if EDTA chelation is the way to hold onto a patient's limb or to snatch the patient from impending death. This book's references may be used by a physician to help him make that decision. That is the purpose for including much scientific and medical material in these next few chapters.

Furthermore, the physician who has his or her curiosity aroused might also interview some patients who have taken chelation treatments. I have discovered these people to be quite open and cooperative. They want to share their experiences and good fortune with others who may benefit.

In the United States and many other Western countries, arteriosclerosis is the most frequently encountered chronic disease.[1,2,3,4] It is implicated in the death of at least every second decedent of our population. And the ratio of deaths caused by hardening of the arteries is increasing annually. The early onset of this disease in over 60 percent of twenty-one-year-old men was documented by autopsy findings in Korea and Vietnam casualties. [5,6] Nobody is immune to the arterial onslaught.

EDTA chelation therapy can reverse those staggering statistics.

A most comprehensive summary of the derivation and development of EDTA chelation is presented in an article, "EDTA Chelation Therapy for Arteriosclerosis: History and Mechanism of Action," authored by Garry F. Gordon, M.D., and Robert B. Vance, D.O. The article is published in *Osteopathic Annals*, February 1976, Volume 4, Number 2, copyright by Insight Publishing Co., Inc., Alfred J. Arsenault, Publisher, 150 East 58th Street, New York, New York 10022.

The senior author of this comprehensive article, Dr. Gordon, is Chairman of the Board and immediate past President of the American Academy of Medical Preventics (AAMP). He had practiced preventive medicine and nutrition in Sacramento, California until he temporarily left medical practice to devote full time to administer AAMP affairs and to spread knowledge of preventive medical techniques, especially as they involve use of chelation therapy.

Dr. Vance is a member of AAMP, a Fellow of the International College of Applied Nutrition, and a charter member of the International Academy of Preventive Medicine and the Academy of Orthomolecular Psychiatry. Dr. Vance is in general medical practice with an emphasis on prevention in Salt Lake City, Utah.

I interviewed both of these physicians. In fact, Dr. Gordon visited in my home for twenty-four hours in October, 1976, when we engaged in a marathon discussion of EDTA chelation therapy. He supplied a great deal of the published source material used to write this book; he has edited the scientific content of this book for accuracy; and he has written its foreword.

Reasons Why Chelation Treatment Is Not Widespread

In their article and in our interviews the co-authors gave me to understand that the administration of chelation therapy is gradually becoming more common for treatment of arteriosclerosis. A number of published medical papers already attest to that. [7-23]

Along with the considerable interest among physicians who have informed themselves about the therapy, however, controversy also surrounds the use of EDTA in several chronic degenerative disease processes. [24-26] That is unfortunate for many patients. Controversy causes doctors to shrink back from using a remedy. They are fearful of being criticized by their physician peers. Although they don't want to be the last to use some treatment, most doctors do not want to be the first, either.

All the possible mechanisms of action of chelation therapy for producing the observed beneficial effects are still incompletely documented. And this incomplete understanding of why and how it works becomes a useful argument employed by medical opponents of the method. Except for those listed in Chapter Three, there has been insufficient medical interest shown in EDTA chelation by large clinical research institutions. There has, in fact, been no full-scale study of the technique. Such a study is needed and has become one of my goals for writing this book.

When delineations become firmly established, improved chelating agents will undoubtedly be developed. They are likely to decrease the inconvenience, time involved, and cost of repeated intravenous infusions. This inconvenient administration technique and the general lack of familiarity with chelating agents[27] are two additional reasons for the serious delay in the widespread utilization of chelation therapy in medical practice. In the meantime, masses of people will continue to die from hardening of the arteries because the American physician has not been educated to the therapy's mechanisms of effective action.

EDTA Mechanisms of Actions Science Understands

Bruce W. Halstead, M.D., current President of the American Academy of Medical Preventics, has written an extensive work on *The Scientific Basis of EDTA Chelation Therapy*, published by Golden Quill Publishers, Inc., P.O. Box 1278, Colton, California 92324. He told me, "I have now reviewed most of the world scientific literature on EDTA, and I am totally convinced that chelation therapy is on solid scientific ground from the molecular to the clinical level."

Dr. Halstead directed my attention to the fundamental action that takes place when EDTA enters an individual's blood vessels. He said, "We find in the course of about the fourth or fifth decade of an adult living in the United States and in most of the developed countries of the world, where atherosclerosis is running rampant, that there is a steady increase in the calcium component in his blood. Along with this extra calcium there is a decline — a depression — in forty-six of the ninety-eight enzyme systems in his body that are active in one facet or another of arterial metabolism. This extra calcium inevitably must cause hardening of the arteries. However, the EDTA chelate directs its activities to the diffuse ionic calcium, which is the particular component that affects those enzyme systems. As a result of the law of mass action, calcium being a very dominant factor, it comes out in excessive quantities during the process of chelation, in an *in vivo* situation. [*In vivo* means that chemical reactions occur in living organisms.]

"EDTA is able to step in there, run through the arterial lumen, and play two roles. It is an intracellular membrane stablizing agent. It removes metallic ions that serve as catalysts in terms of lipid peroxidation and membrane destruction. This first role is possibly the most significant one that EDTA plays, but we are just beginning to understand it," Dr. Halstead said.

"The second significant role of EDTA chelation we *do* understand quite well. Chelation begins to destroy some of the calcium complexes that are inhibiting the enzyme systems. It corrects the shifted enzyme balance that is producing insoluble calcium substance which piles up during the formation of atherosclerotic plaque in the intima wall. EDTA does this by chelating out the insoluble calcium."

Dr. Halstead offered me a summary of the primary actions of EDTA. They are as follows:

1. EDTA reduces the excess ionic calcium which causes inhibition of the enzyme systems of the arterial wall.
2. EDTA tends to stabilize the intracellular membranes of the cells of the arteries, and thus protects the biochemical integrity of the cells.
3. EDTA assists in maintaining the electrical charge of platelets in the blood stream and thereby reduces clumping and blood clots.

"The end result of ionic calcium build-up," said Dr. Halstead, "is the production of an oxygen deficiency state [hypoxia] which triggers off a vicious biochemical cycle of events leading to cellular dysfunction, molecular alterations, a gradual build-up of atherosclerotic plaques, and finally death.

"This biochemical cycle is a series of interacting events involving a complex of nutritional deficiencies, an excessive build-up of metal ion complexes, an accumulation of polluting toxic agents, physical inactivity, and finally an oxygen deficiency state, which is the end result of atherosclerosis," Dr. Halstead explained. "If you examine the overall picture critically, it readily becomes apparent on a rational biochemical basis as to how EDTA functions in reversing hardening of the arteries. EDTA has only one unique ability and that is to be able to form metal ion complexes — to remove these metals from the body."

How EDTA Actually Works in the Blood

What are the chelating agent's actual clinical mechanics? How does it work to take calcium out of atherosclerotic plaque? How may the artery's narrow lumen be widened? These are but a few of the hundreds of questions I endeavored to answer by checking references and asking authorities.

EDTA first binds with the circulating unbound serum calcium to form a calcium-EDTA complex. Much of this complex is excreted in the kidney and bypasses the normal renal conservation of calcium. Drs. Gordon and Vance confirmed this kidney action in their article. They wrote:

> Approximately 80 percent is cleared through the kidney in the first six hours, and 95 percent in the first 24 hours. Some of the EDTA-calcium complex may dissociate, and calcium is dropped when a metal such as lead or chromium, for which EDTA has a higher affinity, becomes available.

Vance and Gordon went on to explain that the loss of calcium through the kidney produces a transient lowering of serum calcium with a concomitant decrease in serum phosphorus, as well as an increase in serum magnesium. All of these chemical alterations with serum heavy metals are beneficial to the heart muscle's contraction by means of an action potential across the membranes.[28] Also, there is a possible holding in balance of electrons.[29] Altogether, a person experiences a number of improvements in myocardial contraction and generalized advantageous heart function and heart rate from the EDTA chelation mechanism. [11,30,31]

The body's homeostatic mechanisms are trying to return the serum calcium to normal levels. It makes this attempt partly through increasing parathormone levels. The initial calcium loss is replaced from the relatively easily changed calcium states of the body. [32-34] Some of the replacement is provided by metastatic (pathologic) calcium that is deposited in scattered remote tissues including the blood vessel walls. Some of it does also leach from the available surface calcium of the skeletal system.

The human body is capable of replacing calcium into the blood at the rate of 50 mg. per minute. Knowing this physiological fact, up to seven times the accepted dose of EDTA could be given in as little as one-tenth the normal administration time — in fifteen minutes instead of in two and a half hours or more as it is administered now — without serious ill effect. EDTA is obviously quite a safe therapeutic aid. I shall discuss safety of use or any possible toxicity of EDTA further in Chapter Seven.

There is no usual complication with the agent's employment, but if a patient develops *hypocalcemia tetany* with the normal dose, his taking magnesium as a nutritional supplement will correct this.[35] *Hypocalcemia* is an abnormally low level of calcium in the circulating blood and commonly denotes subnormal concentrations of calcium ions. *Tetany* is a disorder marked by intermittent tonic muscular contractions, accompanied by fibrillary tremors, paresthesias, and muscular pains; the hands are usually affected when tetany is present.

The increase in parathormone levels, if frequently repeated, leads to activation of osteoblastic bone activity. *Osteoblasts* are the bone-forming cells that build the osseous matrix. Thus new bone can form during or following the chelation process. Indeed, EDTA chelation stimulates new bone formation.

Bone formation from EDTA use takes place in the following manner: The continued osteoblastic activity, when maintained for sufficient time, continues to remove calcium from the blood serum so that soft-tissue pathologic calcium in plaques continues to diminish in order to meet this need caused by the increased bone uptake of calcium. A therapeutic cycle continues: EDTA takes up serum calcium and disposes of it as waste — parathormone activates bone forming cells — bones grow stronger and require more calcium for their build up — more atherosclerotic plaques give off loosely bound pathologic calcium to satisfy the bone cells' demand — the arteries soften and widen steadily in the process. The beneficial effects of chelation therapy are observed to go on for many months following treatment, since bone formation continues at an increased rate and keeps causing dissolution of metastatic calcium.

The late Carlos P. Lamar, M.D., F.I.C.A., one of the original pioneers of calcium chelation in atherosclerosis, had described the reduction in visible aortic calcification with simultaneous apparent recalficication of previously osteoporotic vertebral bones. *Osteoporosis* is a porous condition characterized by scanty, thin and reduced skeletal tissue. [15,18,19] He mentioned seeing improved joint function as arthritic joint calcium deposits are decreased. For that reason, symptoms of arthritis are dissipated. The deformity in a joint may remain, as with Nick Jurich, but mobility returns and pain goes away.

Another advantageous side effect of the chelation mechanism, the strengthening of bones and teeth, can be explained in this way: As reversal of hardening of the arteries takes place, bones and teeth get stronger, because ionic and metastatic calcium that may have avoided being grasped by the chelation claw go into reinforcing existing bone. Thus, hardened arteries get softer and softened bones and teeth get harder from EDTA chelation therapy.

Chapter Five

Additional Internal Actions of EDTA Chelation

The medical importance of chelating agents hinges on the fact that metals play many critical roles in the life of living organisms. In the human body metabolism depends not only on sodium, potassium, magnesium and calcium, but also to a considerable degree on trace amounts of iron, cobalt, copper, zinc, manganese and molybdenum. On the other hand, certain other metals, even in minuscule amounts, are highly toxic to the body. It is apparent, therefore, that chelate drugs with appropriate properties could play several different therapeutic roles. Various chelating agents might be designed (1) to seek out toxic metals and bind them in compounds that will be excreted, (2) to deliver essential trace metals to tissues or substances that require them and (3) to inactivate bacteria and viruses by depriving them of metals they need for their metabolism or by delivering metals to them that are harmful. All three of these hopes have been realized.
— Jack Schubert,
Scientific American, 1966

Chelation Therapy Smooths Skin Wrinkles
Charles H. Farr, M.D., Ph.D., medical director of the Metabolic Disease Center of Norman, Oklahoma, noticed that after treating several hundred patients with chelation therapy, these people appeared to grow younger. Dr. Farr surmised that the mechanisms through which chelation helps the arterial system are essentially the same for the rest of the body. Skin changes that give a younger appearance certainly could occur. Internal actions of EDTA chelation have a relationship to the elastic tissue and collagen tissue in skin.

Elastic tissue, or *elastin,* is the major connective tissue protein of elastic structures such as in large blood vessels and the skin. It affords these structures the ability to stretch, yield to change, and then resume shape or size.

Collagen is the major protein of the white fibers of connective tissue, cartilage, and bone. It has a tendency to overcome the effects of elastin.

One of the factors of aging is that there is a gradual loss of elastic tissue with a build-up of collagen tissue. Thus there is a hardening effect not only of the blood vessels but of the skin and other organs as well.

Patients who have been chelated do remark about changes that they notice in their skin. It becomes smoother — appears much younger than before — wrinkles disappear to a degree.

In order to document these skin changes, Dr. Farr has taken thousands of photographs of patients before and after chelation therapy. Also he has made microphotographs (pictures of skin sections visualized under the microscope). A few of his photographs appear on these pages.

Photograph Six A shows a patient with crows feet at the corner of the eye. The crows feet furrows were wrinkled deeply at the time of photographing, which was August 12, 1974.

Photograph Six B, the same eye area, photographed October 8, 1975, shows the skin remarkably improved in appearance after chelation therapy. It looks younger, smoother, much healthier, and with a loss of wrinkles. This finding, which occurs in some people very rapidly and in others a little slower, is quite consistent.

Photograph Seven A shows Mr. H. W., Dr. Farr's patient, whose "on-face" view pictures the corner of his eye close-up, taken May 2, 1974.

Photograph Seven B of Mr. H. W. shows the same view with a change in his skin folds and wrinkles, taken August 3, 1974 after the man underwent a series of EDTA chelations.

Microphotographs of Skin Biopsies Depict Calcium Deposits

"I was not sure what was accounting for these skin changes," Dr. Farr said, "and this led me to begin doing skin biopsies in order to correlate them with changes in the cellular components themselves. I found two very significant changes that I could document."

The changes illustrated by microphotographs made from Dr. Farr's biopsies are shown in Photographs Eight A, Eight B, Nine A and Nine B. Photographs Eight A and Eight B are stained specifically to depict calcium deposits in the skin before and after chelation therapy.

The microphotograph taken before chelation, *Photograph Eight A* (top), shows the subcutaneous, or fatty muscular layer that lies below the skin, at the upper portion of the photograph, and the larger, well-demarcated darker cells make up the cutaneous, or skin layer, at the lower portion of the photograph.

Compare Photograph Eight A to Photograph Eight B (bottom). Note that the metastatic calcium (the calcium in excess of what the body requires) is heavier, coarser, and more granular. In the loosely bound, relatively non-cellular areas of the upper parts of *Photograph Eight B* it is much less, which indicates that chelation therapy has removed the excessive calcium from the skin. This photograph correlates with the pictures of skin wrinkles before and after chelation.

Dr. Farr said, "I also found that along the basement layer of skin there is some type of fatty tissue or fatty deposit unidentified as yet." In *Photographs Nine A and Nine B* you will see an alteration in the extent of these fatty

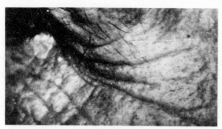
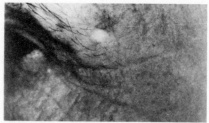

Chelation therapy can smooth skin wrinkles, as these before-and after photographs reveal. *Photograph 6A* shows a patient with crow's feet, but after chelation *(Photograph 6B),* these furrows are remarkably improved.

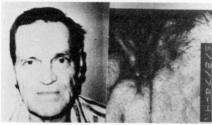
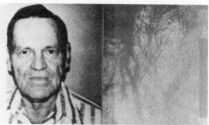

Another exhibit by Dr. Charles H. Farr, showing patient H.W. in *Photograph 7A* (left) prior to treatment and *Photograph 7B* after chelation. Again, the furrows are shallower and the skin is clearer and younger looking.

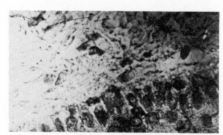
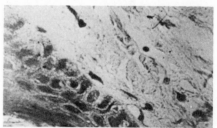

Microphotographs of skin biopsies show the presence of calcium deposits *(Photograph 8A, left)* before chelation therapy and the removal of the heavier, more granular material *(Photograph 8B)* after chelation treatment.

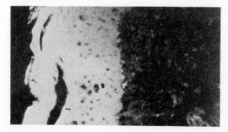
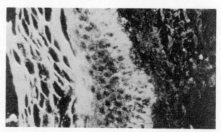

The white and milky materials in *Photograph 9A* (left) are fatty deposits in the outer skin layer, while *Photograph 9B* depicts the same biopsied skin area after chelation.

deposits before and after chelation therapy. These fatty deposits, the white and milky material shown, has something to do with the age and texture of the skin.

Microphotographs *Nine A and Nine B* depict a biopsy slice right through the skin itself with the dark area (at left) being the outside layer of the skin. Comparing these before and after Photographs of Nine A and Nine B, note that chelation therapy in the "after" picture (below) has greatly reduced the white fatty material. Whatever fatty deposits remain run only along the bottom of the basal cell layer of skin.

"From these studies of literally thousands of biopsies and microphotographic views of skin folds, we can deduce that reduction of metastatic calcium deposits have increased the health status of the skin," Dr. Farr said. "The same improved health status should be reflected throughout the entire body because the internal actions of EDTA chelation affects every cell in the body and not just the skin."

Additional Mechanical Actions of EDTA Chelation

In their *Osteopathic Annals* article[1] Dr. Gordon and Dr. Vance told of additional internal results from EDTA chelation. Some of the effects do occur quickly following intravenous infusion. They are likely to be the cause of exceedingly dramatic changes in severely involved people. Although not limited to the mechanical actions which I will describe now, the following benefits also occur:

Calcium is reduced in extracellular fluid, and this is among the most important benefits of the EDTA internal action. The reduction produces a decrease in intracellular free calcium ions that lessens smooth vascular muscle tone or contraction. The result will be the arrest or relief of spasms as in multiple sclerosis or in convulsions as in epilepsy.[2]

EDTA Infusion Has a Mild Pain-Killing Effect

EDTA may work in a way similar to papaverine. *Papaverine* is a non-narcotic drug with a mild analgesic action. EDTA causes analgesia through an inhibition of phosphodiesterase enzyme.[3]

Phosphodiesterase enzyme produces an increase in the concentration of cyclic adenosine monophosphate (AMP), an enzyme, resulting in increased breakdown of glycogen to glucose for easier and more effective sugar utilization by the body.

EDTA Infusion Enhances the Effects of Medication

EDTA medication is directly administered into the vascular compartment by intravenous injection. This infusion produces effective tissue drug levels far above those obtained with oral medication. There is consequent potential for medication effects far superior to those obtained with known oral vasodilators.

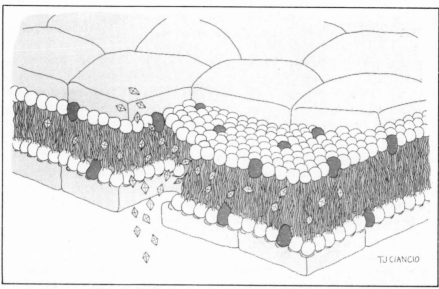

The protective mechanism of EDTA is shown in this illustration of a cell membrane which has been invaded by a toxic divalent mineral (the diamond-shaped particles). When EDTA gets near such a damaged membrane, it binds with the toxic divalent mineral, such as cadmium, lead, tin, mercury, calcium, or zinc. The chelating agent grasps the destructive divalent metal and pulls it out of the membrane; ultimately both the EDTA and the toxic mineral are excreted by the kidneys. Meanwhile, the cellular membrane is coated by enzyme systems, interspersed with beneficial coenzymes such as vitamin E and selenium. Thanks to EDTA chelation, a sick cell has become a healthy one.

Lysosome Functions Like the Toilet of the Body

Intracellular lysosome function may have been impaired by the accumulation of intracellular heavy or toxic metals over the years at the lysosomal membrane. Chelation therapy cleans from the lysosome an accumulation of unwanted waste which may be impairing lysosomal function. In explanation, compare the function of the lysosome in our cells to the action of a toilet in the home. The lysosome helps to flush a cell of its waste products. When toxic trace metals such as lead, mercury, cadmium [5,6] or excess levels of calcium or zinc[7] block the lysosomal membrane, the function of the lysosome will be blocked, too. Blockage contributes to the development of many chronic degenerative diseases such as arthritis, multiple sclerosis, lateral sclerosis, parkinsonism, and more.[8] Removal of these heavy metals will allow the lysosome (the cell septic system) to detoxify more efficiently — even to improve myocarditis due to lead poisoning.[9]

In Chapter Two, I described EDTA as a "chemical rotary snake" that pushes out arterial blockage, or in effect clears the human "pipes." The lysosome is where the metaphor proves itself. Any toilet that becomes stopped-up begins to back up. Like a septic system, lysosomal membranes that are blocked cannot get rid of toxic materials. Because EDTA is an amino acid, it does not just float in the bloodstream, but it also profuses through the tissues, the capillary bed, and in the tissue fluids, pulling out toxic metals from the sixty trillion cells of the body. When EDTA gets near a cellular membrane it binds with any toxic divalent mineral, which is a heavy metal such as lead, tin, mercury, and others that are impairing membrane function and contributing to free-radical damage and lipid peroxidation of these important cellular membranes. The chelating agent pulls out that toxic mineral. Toxins are then floated from the cell by osmosis because there is a greater concentration inside the cell than outside, and that toxin eventually will be excreted from the kidneys. EDTA, therefore, is a membrane stabilizer which works differently than vitamin E and is potentially more powerful.

Why Calcium Is Affected More than Other Serum Minerals

The reason that EDTA is such an effective chelating agent for calcium is because of the wonderful way that nature organized things. The pH of the bloodstream is 7.2 to 7.4. The disassociation curve of minerals with EDTA shows that the mineral most commonly available in the pH range of 7.2 to 7.4 is calcium. Calcium is present in greater amounts than anything else. EDTA takes out lead, mercury, cadmium, zinc, magnesium, manganese, and many other divalent minerals, but calcium seems to form the major metallic complex with EDTA at the normal pH of the bloodstream.

Harold W. Harper, M.D. explained to me that EDTA chelation is virtually an exchange process. "Calcium not only comes off the atherosclerotic plaque. It also affects the calcium pool in the body," Dr. Harper said. "If the physician injects into his patient *dicalcium* EDTA, he will primarily cause an exchange ion or removal of the next heaviest element, which is *lead*. If he injects disodium EDTA, it will exchange with the next higher element at that pH level, which is *calcium*. That is why we inject *disodium* EDTA rather than dicalcium EDTA. The sodium will apparently remain intact in the EDTA molecule and leave the body without increasing the salt load. One of the first and certainly the most prevalent divalent elements EDTA comes in contact with will be calcium. It will bind with that mineral at the bloodstream's 7.2 to 7.4 pH and move toward the kidneys for excretion as calcium EDTA," Dr. Harper explained.

Additionally, I learned from conversations with Garry F. Gordon, M.D. that if the calcium EDTA is allowed by the body to recirculate, it will combine with the next higher mineral in the electromotive series (the periodic table of elements) with highly predictable stability constants. These minerals, which are toxic, include cadmium, mercury, and particularly lead. EDTA in the recirculated calcium form removes the toxic minerals from the body as waste.

Special urine tests such as the twenty-four-hour urine analysis for calcium and the Sulkowich test are used to confirm how much calcium is coming out of an individual's body. The degree of unhardening of his patient's arteries is to an extent measurable by the physician in this way.

Thus the primary effects of the EDTA treatment occur within six hours; however, remember I explained in Chapter Four that the chelation mechanism continues long afterward. For instance, the bones and teeth get stronger because metastatic calcium is absorbed into them over time. Once the process is initiated, therefore, additional excessive metastatic calcium, and other heavy toxic elements, continue to be removed from the lysomal and other cellular membranes.

EDTA Infusion Helps Adjust the Zinc-Copper Ratio

One of the most important ratios in avoiding coronary heart disease is the zinc-copper ratio, which EDTA specifically helps adjust. It improves lipid metabolism, too.[7]

In addition, many enzyme systems become reactivated. Some of these reactivated enzyme systems themselves then work more efficiently to repair damage in the body. Metabolism within the cells functions more normally with this increased cellular efficiency. EDTA acts in this way as a catalytic agent within the body to help make it more able to bring itself into its own desirable balance — known as *homeostasis*. That is why the initial improvement often seen clinically at the time of chelation is not the only effect. The benefits from EDTA infusion continue for sixty to ninety days afterward and occasionally the maximum improvement is seen even beyond ninety days. This is what Dr. Halstead explained in Chapter Four as the first and most significant role played by EDTA. It is this function as an *intracellular membrane stabilizing agent* that provides the optimum beneficial effects. Dr. Halstead called EDTA "an amazing substance for human betterment."

EDTA Chelation Has an Anti-Aging Effect

The incidence of aging is slowed down by EDTA infusion. One of the reasons for this to occur is that EDTA alters tryptophan metabolism.[10] *Tryptophan* is an amino acid component of proteins, which when lowered in bodily content, extends the life span of an individual. This is an anti-aging effect of EDTA chelation which should be investigated by gerontologists. In the book *Prolongevity* (Alfred A. Knopf, 1976), author Albert Rosenfeld suggests that, in time, we can slow the rate of aging, alter the biological clock that may be built into our cells, give our lives a kind of biological daylight saving time, with more sunlight at the end. Science writer Rosenfeld reviewed and explained a great deal of research, but the ultimate technical marvel for slowing aging is with us already, and he overlooked it. EDTA chelation therapy is a gerontologist's rose garden in full bloom.

Plaque Particles Dissolve at Their Tops

If microscopic particles of calcium are uniformly dispersed in atherosclerotic plaque, the EDTA grasps them rapidly.

Dr. Harper told me, "Plaque particles come off not at the base of the plaque but at the top where the bloodstream's eddying currents come in contact with it. Plaque does not project into the lumen like a mountain top but rather like a molehill. Since EDTA attacks plaque where the eddying currents touch, dissolution takes place at the plaque's 'molehill' top where it projects into the lumen to narrow the tunnel that allows blood flow through that artery."

On the other hand, my investigations revealed that if the particles are macroscopic and irregularly dispersed, the calcium will be removed slowly, owing to the particle's small surface-to-volume ratio. [11-15] This probably is one of the reasons that some patients are helped more quickly than others. Their problems are caused by small-size calcium particles; while other patients are more resistant to help and a few may eventually require some direct intervention in the form of surgery for localized blockages that respond too slowly to the infusions of EDTA. Incidentally, the same patient may show both types of calcium deposits, microscopic and macroscopic, even in the same blood vessel, so that many areas in the body having both types of calcium deposits are helped.

Two instruments that measure blood circulation or volume — the *thermogram*, a regional temperature map of the body obtained without direct contact by infra-red sensing devices, and the *plethysmogram*, a recording of the volume of blood flow in a body part or organ — show that capillary bed perfusion is markedly improved by EDTA chelation. Probably this happens at least partially as a result of lowered blood viscosity as well as lowered serum lipids. [13]

Lowering the lipids contributes to decreasing the rouleaux formation by the red blood cells. *Rouleaux* is the stacking or clumping together of these red blood cells just like coins rolled into a wrapper. EDTA has been shown to decrease red cell aggregation (rouleaux). This reduced aggregation speeds blood circulation. Also, decreasing aggregation may be its source of direct benefits to the red blood cells by decreasing the rigidity of their cell membranes. The improved capillary bed perfusion as well as improved peripheral blood flow could also come from the decreased resistance in the blood vessels[16] and other vascular structures induced by the decalcification of elastic tissues with associated decrease in cross-linkages in these tissues. [17-19] Improved capillary bed perfusion could occur additionally from what Gus Schreiber, M.D. of Dallas, Texas described in an unpublished paper[20] — the decrease in basement membrane thickening, particularly in diabetics. Dr. Schreiber performed electron microscope studies of thigh muscle biopsies before and after these biopsied patients underwent chelation therapy.

Rheumatoid Arthritis Symptoms Reduce or Disappear

In the last chapter I described the elimination of Nicholas Jurich's rheumatoid arthritic symptoms. This may be from collagen tissues having their synthesis augmented by the high parathormone levels. Higher parathormone levels, you may recall, are produced in response to the abnormally low levels of calcium in the circulating blood due to the binding of serum calcium by EDTA and its subsequent elimination through the kidneys. Rheumatoid arthritis and other collagen diseases are involved with degradation of mucopolysaccharide and protein connective tissues. Parathormone alters the turnover of these tissues and thus affects rheumatoid arthritis pathology.[21]

Chelation Can Prevent Arthritis

Parathyroid stimulation by EDTA chelation alters the turnover rate of mucopolysaccharides and protein connective tissue components, as I described above.[22] This is important because mucopolysaccharide is a complex of protein and sugar, which when disordered in metabolism causes diseases that include various defects of bone, cartilage and connective tissue. Arthritis of various types will be the result.

By altering membrane calcium components, EDTA chelation increases red blood cell membrane flexibility.[20,23] Greater flexibility allows the red blood cells to fold more easily to conform to the tiniest of capillaries, which may be even smaller than the cells themselves. As a result, *sickle cell anemia* has been reported in the journal *Hospital Practice* to improve from EDTA injection because of the reduced cell wall rigidity.[24] Less rigidity also permits potassium to enter into the cells more readily.[25,26]

High Blood Pressure is Lowered

For a variety of reasons, administration of EDTA chelation lowers the patient's blood pressure levels. This may come from increased excretion of cadmium from kidney tissue cells,[27] the decreased peripheral resistance[16] through increased resiliency of blood vessels after removal of calcium [17-19] and decreased vascular spasm. Moreover, reduced hypertension takes place from increased serum magnesium that I previously mentioned.[28]

EDTA Protects the Liver

EDTA infusions protect against cirrhosis or impairment of liver function in high-fat diets.[23] I already said that it improves lipid metabolism,[29,30] but it also enhances glucose metabolism in diabetic patients.[31,32]

EDTA Chelation Alters Elastin Cross-Linking

EDTA chelation alters cross-linking of elastin, the major connective tissue protein of elastic structures.[17,18] In large blood vessels and elsewhere elastin is a yellow, elastic fibrous mucoprotein. This elastic alteration happening in the aorta has profound consequences, since this cross-linking of mac-romolecules by free radicals and calcium is now thought to be a basic aging mechanism.[33]

Assures the Presence of Adequate Zinc

By means of its binding with zinc, EDTA chelation assures more adequate levels of crucial unstable zinc.[35] Three components — the lactate dehydro-genase enzyme (LDH) of skeletal muscle and nicotinamide adenine dinucle-otide enzyme (NAD) involved in degrading lactate and priming the change of glycogen into glucose, and any damaged cardiac muscle — are improved in their "demand-adaptation" by this change in zinc status.[36]

Offers Psychological Relief

After having no viable approach for relief of significant illnesses, the medical profession now has available EDTA chelation. It is a therapy highly acceptable by patients. Not only does it bring physiological benefit but psychological comfort as well. This psychologic relief is destined to be the cause of removing people's anxiety about dying or losing a limb or an organ. Lowering anxiety levels is proven already, [37,38,39] with resulting vasodilation similar to that taught in "hand-warming" in biofeedback training.

Chelation Therapy Reduces Insulin Requirements for Diabetics

The war inside our arteries against atherosclerotic pathology continues without surcease. Every time another infusion with EDTA is given, more beneficial actions occur — more battles against arterial hardening are being won. To illustrate, insulin requirements are reduced temporarily and good control may be obtained in some diabetics simply by extending this ac-tion through repeated infusions at appropriate monthly or bimonthly intervals. [31,35]

Diabetes mellitus has a well-known relationship to atherosclerosis that is of great importance in chelation therapy. In a study of a large group of patients with atherosclerosis who were without clinical features of diabetes, 56 percent were found to have latent disturbances of carbohydrate metabolism. The insulin disturbances were highest among those with ad-vanced coronary artery heart disease.

In Dr. Norman E. Clarke's series of many thousands of patients with advanced forms of occlusive vascular disease, those with diabetes mellitus responded best to chelation therapy. Dr. Clarke told me that there has been a great reduction in insulin requirements among his patients. He checks their insulin needs frequently and lowers them gradually to avoid a severe insulin crisis. Other chelating physicians have repeated this same observation.

A reduced insulin requirement among diabetics taking chelation therapy has a speculative cause. The role of the pancreas in occlusive vascular disease with its insulin production may also include its islet cells as the source of elastase and its influence in medial elastin metabolism.

EDTA Manages Hyperlipidemia
Plasma lipid levels decrease by an average of 33 percent [7,36,37] so that long-term hyperlipidemias are more easily managed.

Arterial Walls Become More Flexible
Elasticity is restored to rigid, non-stretchy arterial walls. Dr. Clarke explained that the cholesterol in the atheromatous plaque is the product of prior degenerative reactions within the arterial wall. There is thickened fibrocollagenous tissue producing localized intimal enlargement at points of excess hemodynamic stress. Dr. Farr pointed this out earlier in this chapter when he illustrated the formation of skin wrinkles. The collagen deposition antedates the increase in local lipids within the arterial wall. The local intimal enlargements arise from what has been thought were stimulated fibroblasts. More recently, however, it has been demonstrated to be mutant daughter cells from the medial smooth muscle cell proliferating expressly — described as the "monoclonal hypothesis."

Restoration of Media Elastic Tissue
Medical investigation of human aortas has demonstrated alteration in the medial elastic tissue with calcium content increased prior to the appearance of any atherosclerotic plaque. An abundance of mucopolysaccharides in the arterial ground substance serves as fibrillar cement, and enzyme inhibitors of proteolyses that are present in young arteries and permit restoration of arterial wall injury. In older arteries this restoration process is much reduced, but EDTA chelation seems to allow for its return and rejuvenation, through restoration of enzyme function.

At the beginning of this chapter Dr. Farr also demonstrated the reversing of the cross-linking of elastin associated with aging.

There are largely non-sulfated mucopolysaccharides in the arterial wall that decrease with age while the sulphated mucopolysaccharides increase. I learned from Dr. Clarke that sulphated mucopolysaccharides consist chiefly of chondroitin sulphate that has a high affinity for calcium. In the biologically aging artery a change occurs in certain colloids with splitting and fragmentation of elastic fibers.

A group of arteriosclerotic people were found to have a mean yield of nine elastase units while another group of young people (who died through violence) had an average of 208 elastase units. Elastase, like insulin, is formed in the pancreas.

More Lives Saved in Intensive Care and Emergencies
EDTA chelation is projected by Drs. Gordon and Vance to have lifesaving advantages for patients in intensive-care facilities. More people will leave

those facilities alive through the use of this intravenous agent while they are present in the hospital.

EDTA chelation offers protection against the precipitation of lipoproteins that are produced by heparin. *Heparin* is the complex anti-coagulant principle which prevents platelet agglutination and thrombus formation. Precipitation happens in the presence of divalent metals such as calcium. [40,41] Heparin is commonly used during acute heart attacks as crisis care, sometimes without the emergency physician recognizing the danger of increasing ischemia. *Ischemia* is the local lack of oxygenated blood, which is an anemia, due to mechanical obstruction to the blood supply of the heart. *Ischemia* also is defined as a necrosis (death) of a section of the heart through precipitation of prebeta lipoproteins in the presence of stress hormones.[42] By binding calcium and other divalent cations, EDTA chelation can prevent this heparin lipid-precipitation and improve cardiac arrhythmias (irregularities of the heart beat) as well. [25,26]

EDTA Infusion Dissolves Small Thrombi

Another important benefit of the internal EDTA chelation mechanism is the dissolving of small thrombi while the chelating agent is being injected. Dr. Olwin suggested in his presentation in Chapter Three that this benefit does take place. The lowered serum calcium produced by the infusion provides less likelihood of abnormal clotting. To prolong these benefits, the infusions could be given more slowly, such as over a twelve-hour period rather than the two-and-a-half to six hours that they are given now (see Chapter Seven for the method of administration).

Other Diseases Become Treatable

Chelation therapy holds out the promise of success for treatment of various other diseases, as well. These include arthritis, [21,22] porphyria,[40] renolithiasis (kidney stones),[41] scleroderma,[42] lead poisoning,[43] calcium and certain other metal poisonings.[44] I have already emphasized that hypertension is helped. [16,27] There is improvement or restoration of vision in macular degeneration of the retina, as in the case history that Drs. Sibyl and Leon Anderson revealed.

Physicians who employ chelation therapy for vascular occlusive disease, some of whom have joined together in the American Academy of Medical Preventics (AAMP), find that their patients experience a remarkable return of function, in addition to relief of symptoms. The statistical over-all probability of significant improvement of patient functions has been calculated at better than 80 percent.[45] This AAMP combine of enlightened doctors may in time overcome the widespread resistance to such therapy.

Chelation Maintenance Is Important

Often the patients voluntarily return after one or two years for a short series of chelation infusions to prevent any loss of benefits they enjoy. They understand that the arteriosclerotic process is an ongoing degeneration of arterial walls. Our bodies constantly skirmish with this deteriorating disease. Knowing this, some people feel so gratified with their health improvement, having previously suffered severely from ill-health, that they continue to add to their total number of chelation treatments over the years.

There does not appear to be any limit to how many repeat infusions can be taken. [14,29,45] Individuals have received over 500 infusions in a ten-year period; and where the medical history had shown several strokes or myocardial infarctions before chelation with EDTA, they frequently have had no further events during this extended treatment time.

Some, who have full knowledge of chelation advantages, employ the EDTA therapy for other things: a program of illness prevention in advance of any health problem developing, as had Dr. Warren E. Levin (described in Chapter Three); or a preparedness procedure for improved post-operative healing when major surgery is scheduled for the near future, as had Dr. Oswald B. Deiter, whom I shall describe in the next chapter.

Thus, sclerosis of the heart and blood vessels now no longer has to be the end product of the human body's war against our deteriorated environment. Dr. Harper said that the theoretical and practical mechanism for reversal of hardening of the arteries is what we have needed. That mechanism is now available — EDTA chelation therapy. We, who are potential victims of hardening of the arteries, should consider putting it to use immediately. Physicians can acquire the necessary materials and may use the method to offer their patients a virtually nontoxic therapy with potential life-extension benefits. To do this, the technique for administration of EDTA must be understood by both the beneficiary and the benefactor — the patient and the doctor. I shall provide the details of this technique's total method of administration in Chapter Seven. However, first you need to know in advance about the make-up of the ingredients that you might have infused into your blood vessels. I will therefore furnish information about the EDTA solution components next. Let us look at the materials included in the infusion bottle.

Chapter Six

The Uses and Occurrences of EDTA Chelation

Although it is difficult to estimate the extent to which chelating agents are used in treatment of heavy metal poisonings, use of these agents have become the therapy of choice in a number of them . . . . So well established has this form of therapy become that, by and large, uncomplicated cases involving the use of these agents for more commonly seen metal poisonings, i.e., lead, are no longer reported in the literature.
— Harry Foreman, Ph.D.
Federation Proceedings on the Biological Aspects of Metal Binding, 1961

EDTA Chelation as a Pre-operative Preparation

Oswald B. Deiter, D.O. of Ridgewood, New Jersey describes himself as a practicing "ten-fingered osteopath." I recorded an interview with Dr. Deiter aboard an airplane as we flew back from a semi-annual meeting of the International Academy of Preventive Medicine. It was September 12, 1976, two months prior to an operation Dr. Deiter was planning to undergo on his left knee and about one month after he had completed three weeks of daily chelation therapy administered to him by H. Ray Evers, M.D. The patient had made EDTA chelation a part of his preparation for the operation. It was a precaution he had evaluated carefully and elected to adopt.

Dr. Deiter's knee was shot through with osteoarthritis from recurrent injuries. Football once was his forte in college, he told me, but knee trauma which he had sustained then caused the osteopathic physician to suffer now. Additionally, Dr. Deiter had horses fall on him on three separate occasions over the years when he rode to the hounds. His knee condition was much aggravated. To overcome the pain, the physician was scheduled to have a plastic and metal prosthesis inserted into the left knee joint.

Where once this man had been very active in sports, now in his late sixties he sometimes required a wheelchair to get around. An ardent fisherman with a twinkle in his eye, a dry wit, a good sense of humor, and an upbeat outlook, Dr. Deiter longed to become vigorous and sprightly once again. Having the knee surgery might accomplish that, he believed.

The knee operation was carried out November 17, 1976 at the Harkness Pavilion, Columbia Presbyterian Hospital, New York City. To insure quick healing through improved circulation, Dr. Deiter had taken precautionary pre-operative therapy with chelation. Whether chelation treatment really did stimulate faster post-operative repair, the patient has no way of knowing for certain. When I talked to him again in February 1977 he said, "I can tell you that surgery got rid of my degenerative arthritis problem, and I'm completely free of arthritic pain now. I can't prove that chelation helped me to heal more effectively — there's no way to measure — but I suspect it did. The treatment didn't do anything to actually repair my left knee, but now I don't need a wheelchair to get around anymore."

The osteopath also had prepared himself with other pre-operatives. Well in advance of surgery, for instance, he built up his body with heavy doses (megadoses) of vitamins and chelated minerals, especially chelated zinc. *Zinc* is prescribed as a nutrient for patients by alert physicians and surgeons before and after optional surgery because it is known to speed healing.

I persisted and questioned Dr. Deiter about his observed results with chelation, either on himself or on others. "My general body condition improved very much," he answered. "I took chelation to clean out as much atheromatous plaque as possible from my arteries, and I've observed changes in myself which proved that this happened. My blood pressure reduced from 160/110 to 130/70, and it has remained at that level. I showed rather pronounced varicosities in both legs before chelation treatment, but now I've lost the varicose veins in my left leg and about 60 percent of them in the right leg.

"I had trouble previously with moving my right hand due to arthritic problems and old injuries," said the osteopathic physician, "but now I have complete movement of my right hand — no limitation from traumatic arthritis anymore. On this right hand, also, I have what has been labeled a skin cancer. Two years ago the dermatologist wanted to cut it out. I didn't proceed with the skin surgery — just kept the area covered with a vitamin E ointment. Since I've had intravenous chelation, that skin cancer has almost disappeared from my right hand. It is gradually clearing up."

Chelation Results the "Ten-Fingered Osteopath" Observed in Others

Dr. Deiter described a woman he observed at Dr. Evers' clinic. She had been confined at separate times in two nationally known hospitals. Hardening of the arteries of the brain and body had affected her ability to speak and to walk. "She could do neither," he said. His description implied that the woman looked like a Dachau concentration camp prisoner. She weighed less than 89 pounds.

"After having one week of intravenous chelation," said Dr. Deiter, "I heard the woman begin to utter noises. At the end of two weeks she carried on a haltingly soft conversation. In three weeks she was marching around the clinic lobby talking with anyone who would listen. She gained weight and filled out. Her two sons, who alternated weeks staying with her, took her for long walks and other forms of exercise. I watched these really astounding changes take place in that patient and in others from chelation therapy."

The "ten-fingered osteopath" concluded our interview with the description of a second dramatic case. A forty-six-year-old woman from Texas had been brought to the Evers clinic by her husband. "She had been quite active in her church and community," Dr. Deiter explained. "She had been a loving wife and mother and an excellent homemaker, her husband told me, but now she was absolutely demented. She failed to recognize her husband or her grown children or her friends. Suddenly she had gone out of her mind from something affecting her cranial arteries — some dementia. Then Dr. Evers found out the cause. A hair analysis performed on her by the medical staff at the clinic found the woman to be supersaturated with mercury — heavy metal toxicity.

"After being given just a week of daily chelation," Dr. Deiter continued, "the patient went through a marked personality change for the better. She regained her senses! Twenty-four-hour urine specimens taken every third day showed that mercury toxin was just pouring out of her in the hundreds of milligrams because of her receiving the EDTA infusions. While she remained to take more treatment, her husband went home to enlist the help of his city's board of health and all of the various shopkeepers and trade persons they dealt with to uncover the source of massive mercury doses that had been poisoning his wife," Dr. Deiter explained.

Original Use of EDTA for Heavy Metal Toxicity

The original use of disodium ethylene diamine tetraacetic acid (EDTA) in the United States, in fact, was for the treatment of heavy metal toxicity. In this country the agent was first applied against lead poisoning in workers employed by a battery factory. Lead, a toxic heavy metal, was removed from the blood stream and other body storage areas of workers by means of intravenous infusion.

EDTA chelation was also of interest to the U.S. Navy to remove lead from the arteries of sailors who absorbed it while they painted the Navy's ships and dock facilities. The therapy is still used for that purpose.

The medical potential of the chelating agent was demonstrated dramatically in 1951 when EDTA saved the life of a child suffering from lead poisoning (see "Chelation," by Harold F. Walton; *Scientific American*, June, 1953).

Physicians observed that patients who had both lead poisoning and arteriosclerosis began to improve exceedingly well following chelation treatments with EDTA. Seeing their vascular conditions change for the better, the doctors started to treat others with vascular conditions who did not have lead poisoning. It was no surprise that patients with just occlusive vascular disease improved, too. In fact, the investigation of the medical uses of chelating agents has produced a voluminous literature, and chelate drugs have been developed for the treatment of a wide range of diseases from metal poisoning to cancer. The latest is for treatment of radioisotope saturation.

Besides citric acid and aspirin, other common chelating agents are cortisone, Terramycin, and adrenalin. There are a host of additional chelating compounds, natural and synthetic, probably numbering in the tens of thousands.

Full Food and Drug Administration (FDA) approval has never been given for EDTA use against occlusive vascular disease, however. Intravenous infusion is the only route used because the chelating substance is poorly absorbed and not readily tolerated when taken by mouth. It does not cross the intestinal membrane well, with only five percent absorbed on the average. The stomach gets upset when EDTA is swallowed in its therapeutic form, although it is a common additive to many foods.

Chelation with EDTA remains an approved method for lead detoxification from the human body. It is excellent for that purpose, and this was confirmed as far back as 1961 during the Federation Proceedings on the Biological Aspects of Metal Binding from which I took the quotation at the beginning of this chapter. Recently, the State University of New York, Downstate Medical Center College of Medicine in Brooklyn, used calcium EDTA to treat hyperactivity of children, with excellent results. The medical authorities there believe that these children may have benefitted because their hyperactivity may have represented an increased susceptibility to lead toxicity. They did not have true "lead poisoning" by accepted definition.

Heavy metal toxicity is much more prevalent throughout the world and even more serious than is commonly recognized.[1] It is apparently more effectively diagnosed with hair analysis[2] than with conventional blood and urine tests.[3] Previously accepted "safe levels" of heavy-metal exposure lately have been found to cause or aggravate many chronic diseases.[4] Hyperactivity in children,[5,6] myocarditis,[7] and neuropathy due to lead[4] and hypertension due to cadmium are among those heavy metal toxicity diseases now recognized. After chelation, repeated hair analysis confirms the decrease in heavy metals as well as the improved trace minerals levels after adequate nutritional supplements are taken. Failure to show these changes may suggest the need for further reevaluation by the chelating physician. The physician will probably look for continued unrecognized heavy-metal exposure, as well as potential absorption or excretion defects in trace mineral metabolism.

Vitamin and Mineral Therapy Is Needed

Zinc and chromium deficiencies are readily diagnosed with hair testing in order to eliminate all potential causes of arteriosclerosis, [1,8,9] as well as to help maintain chelation benefits, and to achieve even greater improvement with the maximum elimination of symptoms. Hair analysis also contributes to greater chelation safety by avoiding potential aggravation of mineral deficiencies (such as zinc and chromium) through early recognition of these increased needs of some patients. Today's chelating physicians minimize the potential for EDTA toxicity by providing appropriate mineral and vitamin therapy along with the intravenous injections. [10,11,12]

Chelation therapy is now known to bind and thus remove certain of the B-complex vitamins, [11] particularly pyridoxine, as well as many essential trace metals, [12,13,14] notably zinc and chromium. It is therefore logical that clinicians using chelation therapy had to become keenly aware of the recent developments regarding the benefits of these vitamins and minerals in arteriosclerosis. [15,16] Mineral therapy and vitamin therapy are integral additions to the chelation therapy program. Hair analysis for evaluation of the patient's trace mineral status is performed routinely. [17-20] The program of treatment against hardening of the artieries, obviously, then, is not confined to EDTA chelation therapy alone. The anti-atherosclerotic program includes suggestions for dietary supplementation, vitamins, chelated minerals, special foods and other items.

Soviet physicians employed a chelator called *Unithiol* with a multivitamin administration in coronary arteriosclerosis. The Russians encourage the use of vitamin and mineral supplements for their people. They cited several sources in their 1973 and 1974 articles regarding the use of vitamins and Unithiol in arteriosclerosis. [24,25] The Soviet medical scientists concluded that such early treatment with dietary supplements and chelation is the most successful anti-coronary approach. They recommend this combination treatment for the prevention of arteriosclerosis in the aging as well. This comprehensive approach of chelation, mineral and vitamin therapies may explain the great success some of today's clinicians are seeing in treating vascular disease. It is truly a "holistic" approach. Other informed and forward-looking doctors are beginning to use these holistic concepts as a more total treatment program for their patient's health problems. It includes nutritional therapy and chelation therapy, among other things.

Varieties of the Chelation Agents

Chelation agents are somewhat like aspirin in that all of the mechanisms by which they exert their beneficial effects are presently still not known. I outlined a number of recognizable benefits provided by EDTA chelation in Chapters Four and Five, but there are probably more as yet unacclaimed.

The Soviet chelating agent that I mentioned, Unithiol, employs a sulfhydryl group as the chelator. [22,23] When combined with orthomolecular nutrition (the use of megadose nutritional supplements) and regular exercise, this approach was so successful that some knowledgeable Russian physicians now use it for an anti-aging procedure. It turns back the clock on the wearing out of tissues and reduces the incidence of hardening of the arteries for many older people.[23] As the foundation principle for reversal of hardening of the arteries, Soviet physicians are providing their patients with an excellent program. A similar program is used in Czechoslovakia.

In 1972, the Czechoslovakian article "Chelates in the Treatment of Occlusive Atherosclerosis"[23] concluded that EDTA was the treatment of choice for vascular disease producing intermittent claudication of the legs.

It should thus be clear that all of us in the Western world have at least four choices by which to govern how and when we might live and die. Until now, only two of these choices have been offered. The choices are: (1) the extreme of simply watching and waiting for the expectant death caused by hardening of the arteries; (2) the other extreme of traditional medicine's totally inadequate "medical" *palliation* for the relief of arteriosclerotic symptoms in whatever organ the disease happens to strike;[24] (3) the intermediate between these of vascular surgery as a life-preserving technique, which consists of rather radical surgical procedures; or (4), what this book shows you as a fourth choice, the preventive and reversal treatment with EDTA chelation and nutritional therapies. Which is the choice selected by you?

Commercial and Medical Chelation Substances

The chemical principle of chelation has been in use for at least a century in many industrial processes. For example, the softening of water is a process of chelation. Certain ion exchange materials, such as zeolite (used to soften water), are chelates. Zeolite is a complex sodium compound. When it comes in contact with hard water, it exchanges sodium for calcium and magnesium, which are the two minerals that make water hard. No lather forms when soap is added to hard water; a scummy precipitate drops out instead. Zeolite chemically forms sodium carbonates and sulfates to provide softened water. That is exactly how EDTA and other chelating agents work.

Chelation also forms the basis for the action of some of the other more commonly used detergents. Just as the chelating physician does for patients, the modern homemaker employs the principle of chelation when she uses detergents to wash clothes and dishes. Detergents form soluble chelates with calcium and magnesium that are readily washed out by water rinsing. That way no scum builds up as a ring around the dishwashing machine, bathtub, or wash basin.

The chelation process is used extensively in modern medicine. In addition to those I have already mentioned, such pharmaceuticals include penicillin, penicillamine, tetracycline, streptomycin, bacitracin, oxytetracycline, polymyxin, ammonia, cyanide ion, glycine, oxine, dipyridyl, tetraethyllithuram, vitamin B-12, isoniazid, aminosalicyclic acid, and many others. Each chelating agent has a varying affinity for a variety of cations, depending upon the various spatial arrangement of the ligand molecule and many additional chemical and physical factors.

For the educational benefit of physicians and physical chemists who are among our readers, I will list a few of the chelating agents used in medicine to directly achieve a desired chelation effect. These chelating agents were made known to me by Paul H. Huff, Ph.D. in his March 1974 presentation to the American Academy of Medical Preventics:

- Diethylenetriaminepentaacetate (DTPA)
- Cyclohexane trans 1, 2-diaminetetraacetate (CDTA)
- Ethylenediaminetetraacetate (EDTA)
- Isopropyllenediaminetetraacetate (IPDTA)
- Bis (-aminoethyl) ether tetraacetate (BAETA)
- (2-hydroxyethyl) ethylenediaminetetraacetate (HEEDTA-N)
- (2-hydroxycyclohexyl) ethylediaminetetraacetate (HCDTA-N)
- Nitrilotriacetate (NTA)
- Ethylenediamine di (0-hydroxyphenylacetate) (EDDHA)
- (2-hydroxyethyl) iminodiacetate (HEIDA-N)
- Di (hydroxyethyl) glycine (DHEG-N, N)
- 2,2-dimethylthiazoladine-4carboxylic acid (DTAC)
- 2,3 dimercaptoproponol (BAL)

The earliest medical therapeutic use for which the chelation principle was applied was with dimercaprol or *British antilewisite (BAL)*, discovered during World War II by Professor R. A. Peters and co-workers in Oxford, England. BAL is an antidote against the vesicant poison gas lewisite. By chelating the three arsenic atoms in the lewisite molecule it renders the gas harmless and easily removable from the skin by water or from the body tissues in the urine. BAL became the first chelating agent used in the routine treatment of arsenic and other metal poisons during the 1940s. Unfortunately, BAL's own irritating effects upon living tissues severely limited its widespread employment. Subsequently, other chelating agents were sought that could be used internally with fewer undesirable side effects. That is why EDTA came into common use for therapeutic purposes.

The Chemical Formula of EDTA

EDTA has been designated by a variety of names by scientists in the papers they have published. Various names given to EDTA have included disodium ethylene-diamine tetraacetate; disodium ethylenediamine tetraacetic acid; edathamil; endrate; edathamil calcium disodium; disodium endrate; Sequestrene; disodium Versenate; triolone-B; disodium EDTA, and perhaps others. Its chemical formula is:

```
O==C—OH                              HO—C==O
   |                                     |
H—C—H                                 H—C—H
   |          H    H                     |
   N——————————C————C——————————————N
   |          |    |                     |
H—C—H         H    H                   H—C—H
   |                                     |
O==C—O—Na                          Na—O—C==O
```

In the presence of a bivalent metallic cation such as calcium, ($Ca =$), each of the two-OH radicals release their hydrogen atom, replacing it with each of the two cation metallic valences thus firmly sequestering the cation within a chelate ring (also see photograph five). Then the formula of disodium EDTA changes to:

```
O==C—O————————Ca————————O—C==O
   |         ⁄    \                    |
H—C—H       ⁄      \                 H—C—H
   |       ⁄   H    H  \                |
   N———————C————C———————N
   |           |    |                   |
H—C—H          H    H                 H—C—H
   |                                     |
O==C—O—Na                          Na—O—C==O
```

The first report of experimental control of serum calcium levels *in vivo* was made by Popovici and co-workers in 1950.[25] In 1951 Rostenberg and Perkins[26] used EDTA topically in the treatment of dermatitis appearing in nickel and cobalt miners. That same year Proescher[27] discovered that EDTA had some anticoagulant properties, leading to the finding of its strong calciotropism. *Calciotropism* is the attraction or grasping quality for calcium cations floating in the blood. More published clinical papers kept coming after that and any search of the medical literature will turn up several hundred clinical papers published during the 1950s.

Research reports came from scientists in Switzerland, Germany, France, England, the United States, Japan, and Australia. The Australian National University, in fact, listed 175 references in 1960. Probably the most attention-demanding papers for our purposes were Dr. Clarke's two reports, published in 1955 and 1956. They gave dramatic descriptions of the successful treatment of vascular disease with the removal of calcium from arteries by intravenous EDTA. Dr. Clarke's papers also told of the correction of an apparently terminal case of uremia, which I discuss in detail in the next chapter. It was in a patient who had progressive nephrocalcinosis (calcification of the kidney), studied by X-ray during its evolution for several years. [28,29]

The Suppliers of EDTA

The Dow Chemical Company has been a supplier of EDTA in the United States since the early 1950s. Ciba-Geigy Corporation, a pharmaceutical firm, later became a supplier of chelation raw materials. Riker Laboratories makes an intravenous injection solution of calcium disodium versenate 9.2 mg. per ml.

Another major drug manufacturer, Abbott Laboratories, began to market EDTA in 1959. Abbott Laboratories had listed vascular occlusive disease as an indication for EDTA therapy for several years, from the time of Dr. Clarke's several published reports and from research reinforcement provided by the late Carlos P. Lamar, M.D. during his striking case presentations made to the American College of Angiology in 1964 and 1968. [30,31]

Some small pharmaceutical companies such as Pharmex, Inc. of Hollywood, Florida, Fellows-Testagar of Detroit, McGuff Company of Burbank, California, and others are now suppliers of EDTA.

EDTA Is No Longer Approved for Occlusive Vascular Disease

Although EDTA is both safe and useful, I must keep the record straight and tell you that Abbott Laboratories has removed all mention of vascular occlusive disease from its package insert. When the Food and Drug Administration asked for substantiation of Abbott Laboratories' claims, under the congressionally imposed Drug Efficacy Regulations, Abbott dropped all those claims relating to occlusive vascular disease. Abbott's reason was strictly financial. The potential required research costs to Abbott were simply too high for the company to hope to recover them in the few remaining years before the EDTA patent rights expired. Consequently, arteriosclerotic diseases are not included as a use for Endrate® on the Abbott Laboratories package insert. Oddly, for reasons no one has fully been able to explain, a comment *against* the use of the drug in "Arteriosclerosis Associated with Advancing Age" remains printed on the Abbott package insert. It is there without any supporting documentation.

Thus today, the physician who wants to offer chelation therapy to his patients has to understand the significance of that now seriously restrictive package insert. The lack of a listed indication for its use in arteriosclerosis puts increased responsibility on the physician to be completely knowledge-able about the medication and how it is to be used.

The American Medical Association (A.M.A.) has recently petitioned the FDA to put a disclaimer on the bottom of *all* package inserts in use for *all* drugs to ease this severely increased physician responsibility. However, physicians regularly utilize drugs in a manner not listed on the package insert. FDA documents point out that this physician practice is both legal and ethical. The FDA has not been instructed by Congress to interfere with the physician's use of a drug.

Again, let me clarify that Abbott Laboratories no longer lists "vascular occlusive disease" under the indications for Endrate® and the statement that "it is not recommended for the treatment of generalized arteriosclerosis associated with advancing age" does appear without any explanation given for its presence.

Abbott's statement about arteriosclerosis in the aging may represent an attempt at legal protection for the company against the drug manufacturer. That probably was done because EDTA toxicity was so poorly understood in the early years of the agent's use. I shall discuss possible toxicity in the next chapter.

Previously, EDTA was indicated on the package insert for angina or peripheral vascular disease when symptomatic disease presented a threat. Any risks of use were outweighed by the benefits in the face of the symptomatic vascular disease process. For simply delaying arteriosclerosis of aging, however, Abbott Laboratories had decided many years ago that the risk appeared too great until new information on toxicity is elaborated. [12, 32-34]

You should be informed as well that this new information about lack of toxicity exists today. But Abbott Laboratories is virtually powerless to change a single word on a package insert without expending millions of dollars to get the FDA to agree. As a reader of this book you may be able to change these "catch-22" situations. New Federal legislation may become necessary to facilitate the widespread availability of some form of chelation therapy for all U.S. citizens who desire it, following appropriate informed consent procedures with their physicians. Yes, public acceptance of this book may help make the difference.

Chapter Seven

Components, Technique, and Toxicity of Administering Chelation

In view of the repeatedly confirmed safety of this therapy and of its possible great benefits in the preservation of usable and enjoyable life and health for the many millions of people affected by calcific atherosclerosis and other calcium metastatic lesions, a concerted study of large numbers of institutional volunteer subjects (in homes for the elderly, in long-term care facilities, and in prisons) should be carried out, with matched controls receiving intravenous placebo solutions. All subjects should be thoroughly studied before and during therapy and for prolonged follow-up periods, by all available means including perhaps vascular biopsy studies. Only a mass investigation of this type can clarify the role of chemical endarterectomy in the prevention, early correction and late palliation of the metabolic disturbances which result from reduced blood supply through arteries with lumens narrowed by atherosclerotic plaques.

— Carlos P. Lamar, M.D.
Journal of the American Geriatrics Society, March, 1966

How to Increase American Life Expectancy

Chelation therapy allows a person with occlusive vascular disease to optimize his response to all the various forms of therapy he takes. As a single-modality approach, EDTA chelation is unsurpassed. It must be combined, however, with a comprehensive, multi-therapeutic approach that includes re-establishment of optimum metabolic equilibrium through diet, exercise, reduced stress and nutritional supplementation. Then there is an unexcelled effect. This is the orthomolecular-holistic approach where occlusive vascular disease processes will be generally controlled and possibly reversed.

All known risk factors for hardening of the arteries must be identified, treated, and eliminated, if possible. For example, defective lipid metabolism must be improved with diet, nutritional supplements, and hormones, instead of the current inadequate practice of surgical expediency or the other extreme of watching and waiting. Look at the prevalent practice of American medicine today — we wait for a crisis after watching a disease pattern take hold. Then we attack the problem — not infrequently using expensive and dangerous surgical procedures. Fortunately, a few enlightened physicians have had the honesty to look at what they are doing and make changes.

Current forms of orthodox American crisis-oriented medicine for hardening of the arteries invariably arrives with too little, too late. And chelation or supplemental nutrition is not even included as one of these orthodox therapies. I believe arteriosclerosis and other forms of chronic, degenerative disease that confront Americans can be reduced and even eliminated through application of these orthomolecular-holistic medical concepts, which is the practice of preventive medicine in its most ideal form.

Holistic medicine holds great validity, for through its practice the number of illnesses that affect all people can be much more effectively controlled — and at far lower costs in lives, dollars, and time.

The intravenous approach for the administration of EDTA has been made a part of the holistic approach. However, this technique to increase every American's life expectancy no doubt can be improved upon. Someday, perhaps, one infusion might do the work of several. This improvement would lower the cost associated with current administration techniques and thus increase the acceptance of the concept, not only for the restoration of blood flow through diseased vessels, but also for the amelioration and prevention of several other disease processes. Until that general acceptance by the people and their physicians occurs, the components, administration technique, and costs of intravenous chelation are not likely to change much. My fear is that acceptance may come too late to have this important therapy included in any forthcoming national health program. If that be the case, its availability to the American people could be seriously threatened by the ever-present red tape of bureaucratic regulations usually associated with government-controlled medicine. [1-7]

Components of the EDTA Solution

The infusion of EDTA is medically simple and the components in the bottle are not mysterious. The infusion solution of EDTA in the form of *Pharmex Cheladrate®* or *Endrate disodium®* (edathamil disodium, Abbott) is supplied in 20-cc ampoules containing 150 mg per ml for a total of 3.0 gm of the drug in each ampoule. It is usually administered by adding the contents of one of these ampoules to a bottle containing 500 ml of lactated Ringers solution or normal saline or 5 percent dextrose aqueous solution. A solution of 10 percent fructose or levulose, an invert sugar, may also be used as the vehicle, especially if the patient is a diabetic. Dr. Lamar has noted that "a high percentage of absorbed levulose is utilized as such by the diabetic patient without the need for additional insulin." Also, the levulose is a better form of liver glycogen than dextrose. [8]

To this solution different physicians add various components for specific purposes in accordance with the patient's needs. Five to 40 cc of procaine aqueous 2.0 percent or Lidocaine 2.0 percent (for intravenous use), which are both local anesthetics, may be added to the 500 cc solution, if necessary. These reduce possible local burning or pain at the injection site that might be connected with intravenous injection. Doctors use a local anesthetic administered intravenously with great caution because a certain percentage of patients may be allergic to these drugs and have some reaction. The pain of infusion from venous spasm is only slight, however, especially if the local anesthetic in the solution is used as needed for comfort control. Lately, it has been found that most people will not require any anesthetic if magnesium sulfate, 2 cc to 4 cc of 50 percent strength, is added to the infusion. Excellent biochemical rationale exists for adding magnesium because of its competitive antagonism to calcium.

Doctors use another control, too. Any pain of solution administration is effectively reduced by lowering the rate of infusion. Usually sixty drops per minute is adequate for a three-to-four hour infusion, and this can be slowed down for a patient who is more sensitive. The solutions which cause the least discomfort seem to be levulose first, dextrose next, then saline, and finally Normosol, which is a product manufactured by Abbott Laboratories. However, with the addition of magnesium, all the solution administrations are essentially pain-free.

Dr. Lamar recommended the additon of 5,000 I.U. of heparin sodium to the solution.[9] Physicians used heparin previously to help avoid thrombophlebitis, which could occur with any intravenous solution. Lately it has been learned that heparin decreases blood viscosity and thus aids capillary circulation, which is highly desirable during chelation. As a rule, therefore, doctors who chelate do put sodium heparin in the bottle.

Vitamin C Nutritional Supplementation

Vitamin C, or ascorbic acid, is frequently included in the bottle, as well. About 7.5 to 12.5 grams of ascorbic acid is made part of the intravenous infusion as a chelation "push." Paul Huff, Ph.D. suggested that vitamin C helps to wipe out the *rouleaux effect* or clumping of red blood cells. A person under stress who is hostile, angry, ill-tempered, or suffers in some other way will have more of a rouleaux effect than the person who is well-adjusted, happy, calm, relaxed, and showing a stable personality. The dark field of the microscope will illustrate this. Acidifying the pH of the blood by adding vitamin C to the chelation solution may clear the blood of signs of stress.

Vitamin C also aids collagen tissue repair which is a desirable feature in arteriosclerosis therapy. Additionally, vitamin C is partially responsible for regulation of cholesterol content of the blood. Biochemist Richard A. Passwater states, "Vitamin C tends to normalize the blood-cholesterol level and consume the cholesterol deposited in the arteries: vitamin C can clear cholesterol from the arteries and cure atherosclerosis."[10]

Additional Oral or Injectible Nutrients

Included in the 500 cc infusion, or added as another intravenous "push" injection later, will be varying dosages of other vitamins and minerals. Often given as a separate injection are vitamin B6, 100 mg; a separate vitamin B complex that contains 150 mg of the many B vitamins such as vitamin B-1, vitamin B-2, choline, inositol, and others; 150 mg of niacinamide (vitamin B-3); 1000 mcg of vitamin B-12; plus 500 mg of vitamin C if it has not been included in the original EDTA solution.

Mineral supplementation in the form of daily tablets or capsules taken at home are a requisite also. EDTA chelation therapy causes depletion of the body stores of zinc, magnesium, iron, and other metals, and they must be replaced by mineral nutrients taken with your meals.

The American medical profession, except for those physicians who practice holistic medicine, fails to recognize the important aspects of orthomolecular nutrition with megavitamin therapy, megamineral therapy, and the optimum diet. Self-treatment with orthomolecular nutrition to reverse hardening of your arteries is a program that fits "hand and glove" with chelation therapy.

The Administration Method of EDTA Chelation

To learn how the complete course of chelation care is administered, I interviewed Warren M. Levin, M.D., F.A.A.F.P., a chelating physician. Dr. Levin said, "I use a modified salt solution as the EDTA infusion vehicle. I don't like to give sugar solution intravenously. In those cases where patients do not tolerate intravenous salt solution well, I will use a fructose solution, since glucose affects the body's insulin levels and fructose does not.

"Thus using a diluting fluid of salt or fructose (a sugar), I infuse about 500 cc, roughly about a pint of solution, to which I have added the correct dose of EDTA, which is usually 20 cc. The dose seldom varies from person to person but remains at three grams per 500 cc of solution," he explained.

"I have been adding heparin to the fluid to help prevent any clotting problems. We know that heparin acts in the last phases of the clotting process where prothrombin becomes thrombin and thrombin reacts with fibrinogen to make fibrin. Fibrin is the material that makes the clot. Heparin inhibits the clot formation. But one of the first steps in clotting is platelet aggregation. Heparin does enhance platelet aggregation. In a sense, then, we're fighting what we are trying to accomplish, and this knowledge has caused me to re-evaluate the addition of heparin to my EDTA intravenous solutions. Up to now my fellow members of the American Academy of Medical Preventics who give chelation therapy incorporate heparin into the infusion solution."

The Intravenous Infusions a Patient Experiences

A patient's experiences with receiving chelation therapy is pleasant, albeit boring, for the first few three to six-hour procedural visits, until he arrives prepared to accomplish some reading and writing during the treatments. I will describe the procedure in minute detail so that you will know what to expect. Also, my description may aid your doctor when he decides to adopt this treatment as part of his practice.

Each visit, you sit in a reclining chair and the procedure will invariably be the same for all of the treatments. The physician, or nurse, acts as "intravenous technician" and attaches a disposable infusion set to the prepared bottle of EDTA solution. An extension tube set and a small vein needle are added. (The needle is labeled set g-21.) The technician fills the tubing with fluid to expel all the air present. A strip of white adhesive tape is affixed alongside the bottle's graduated markings. When the infusion begins the technician writes down the time at each successive 100 cc mark. Each bottle in your series of infusions is numbered in that way.

The doctor or the nurse, as technician, has the option to select a venipuncture site at your ankle, next to the internal (tibial) malleolus on the leg, or along one of your forearms. A site is chosen alongside and preferably above a firm bone surface away from moveable joints and usually not in the hands. This selection thus gives the technician an option to use or not use an infusion board. Your physician or his nurse injects the needle into your limb as part of that office's preferred chelation procedure.

Needle insertion consists of the technician engorging your vein site carefully by massaging and gently slapping the part. Then a small Velcro tourniquet is applied. He or she cleans the skin with alcohol and verifies the fullness of your vein. An assistant to the technician holds the bottle hanging down at a level well below the vein and keeps the bottle valve closed.

Then the technician folds the needle wings together and holds them between thumb and forefinger, the opening upwards and pointing in the direction of the vein's blood flow. The skin and vein wall are punctured in one quick motion that is practically painless. The assistant opens the bottle valve to create suction in the tubing. As blood shows in the tubing, the technician releases the tourniquet, flattens the needle wings, and affixes them with a short strip of transparent microspore adhesive tape.

The technician's assistant raises the bottle very slowly while adjusting the drip valve to about twenty drops per minute at the start. The technician affixes successive coils of tubing to the skin with separate strips of tape. A last piece of tape, long enough to go around, is dropped over the connecting glass segment of the needle set and is draped gently around the limb without pressure. The assistant hangs the bottle in its hook on a stand for that purpose, and the technician writes down the starting time for the infusion on the white tape at zero level.

Patients are observed for a few minutes each time to assure the technician that the infusion is well-tolerated. From time to time the drip rate is adjusted to have it run at slightly faster than one hour for each 100 cc. Five hundred cubic centimeters of solution are administered. The procedure averages four hours a visit, while slower rates may be used for sensitive patients.

Medical Problems Encountered During the Chelation Technique

You will experience few, relatively minor discomforts during the infusions. There might be slight bleeding into the tissue, with some black and blue areas and swelling from the hematomas.

Since the material being infused is somewhat irritating and different people have various levels of sensitivity, it is to be expected that a patient might have discomfort from the solution going through his arm. Side effects could include nausea, vomiting, burning or stinging at the site of infusion, subnormal arterial blood pressure, drops in blood sugar level with subsequent feelings of fatigue, dermatitis, muscle spasm or tetany, and other possible problems. To prevent stinging, the doctor sometimes uses the local anesthetic, procaine, which is added to the intravenous solution.

Another technique to eliminate intravenous sting is to change the solution composition by making an alteration in acidity, alkalinity, magnesium salts, and other means. This reduces infusion discomfort.

I spoke to Dr. Levin about the various problems that he encounters administering intravenous chelation with EDTA. Afterall, any time a needle is introduced into a vein there is the risk of infection.

"That's true," he said, "but, thank God, we've never had any infection. A doctor who puts needles into veins often enough is sure to inadvertently irritate a vein somewhere along the line. There is always the possibility of inducing an inflammation with clot formation, called *thrombophlebitis*. Generally this thrombophlebitis is not the kind of a clot in the vein that breaks off and travels through the circulatory system and produces problems. It is a local inflammatory response to irritation. The body takes care of the inflammation over time. The local thrombophlebitis can be annoying, but it's of no serious consequence to the patient and can occur during any infusion and not just from chelation."

In passing, I'll mention that vitamin E is known to avert this particular problem of local inflammation — or, in large doses, vitamin E seems to speed recovery from local thrombophlebitis.

"If someone is in heart failure or has severe high blood pressure," Dr. Levin continued, "giving extra sodium (which is the main component of the salt solution) intravenously is probably not a good idea. That individual would be one of the patients for whom I might use the fructose solution.

"Furthermore, allergy to one or all of the substances in any infusion is always a possibility. Allergic reactions can be serious enough to warrant temporarily discontinuing the therapy. It has been my good fortune not to have any serious allergic reactions to chelation therapy in this office," smiled the physician.

Dr. Levin added, "If the needle slips out of the vein and fluid seeps into the tissues it can feel painful and irritating, but no significant or long-term harm ensues. The reaction is about like a bee sting.

"Some people do feel a little nauseated during therapy and immediately afterward," he said. "They don't feel well for a day or so after the infusion. They experience non-specific symptoms such as blurred vision and thickened speech that is referable to the changes in calcium levels and an inability of the body to equilibrate itself as it gets older.

Nephrotoxicity of Chelation Therapy

The initial use of EDTA in 1954 was associated with two deaths [11,12] for which serious overdosages of up to 10.0 gm per infusion are blamed. Later, the recommended dose was lowered to 5.0 gm. and then to 3.0 gm.; [13] but it was only after the development and use of the electron microscope and other careful studies that this question of potential toxicity was fully clarified. [14-16] The conclusion of these studies was that the term "nephrotoxic," which Dr. Levin had referred to as "transient kidney malfunction," is *not* justified with EDTA. The change seen in the kidney is a normal physiologic mechanism for removal of toxic products through the kidney. There is *no* long-term damage or development of later kidney complications associated with EDTA when the intravenous technique is properly employed. After all, even water and air can be toxic when applied improperly.

Norman E. Clarke, M.D. wrote a report on the death of one of these EDTA-associated patients. It was in his early investigation of EDTA that one of Dr. Clarke's chelation cases, a sixty-eight-year-old mechanic identified as W. McL., who had his first attack of angina in 1947, might possibly have had his death hastened from a high-dose related EDTA infusion. That was more than twenty-five years ago.

Dr. Clarke stated, "The patient's activities had been unlimited until early 1953. Then he had a diseased gall bladder removed in November, 1953, after which he improved until January, 1954, when angina pectoris increased rapidly."

In February, 1954, Dr. Clarke gave the patient fifteen intravenous injections of 5.0 grams each within less than three weeks (a total of 75 grams). This amount was about three times what is now considered to be the usual and customarily acceptable dosage. A few days later the man had a convulsion, lost consciousness, and died within a few hours. His autopsy disclosed that he also had previously unrecognized kidney disease, which further points out the necessity of first determining kidney function in all patients before they receive chelation.

Dr. Clarke continued with his report: "At necropsy [autopsy] they demonstrated extensive atherosclerosis. In some zones the atheromatous material containing lipid was diminished and in other zones there was necrosis and degeneration of supporting stroma and slight polymorphonuclear infiltration. The coronary arteries section showed intense medial sclerosis with calcification and general narrowing of the lumen, but no atheroma. The kidneys had tubular nephritis and glomerulitis that was considered to be terminal. There was no vacuolization of the kidney cells. The coronary pathology was medial sclerosis with no occlusion or atheroma."

As an interpretation of this medical autopsy report offered by Dr. Clarke, the innocent lay reader should be told that the patient was probably doomed to die momentarily no matter what treatment he received. The disease in the man's kidneys alone could be the cause of his death. Or the mechanic could have died from coronary artery blockage.

As an explanation of that long ago case, Dr. Clarke has said, "That was during the early period when we were giving up to ten grams of EDTA. We didn't know what to give, it being the first use of the compound on atherosclerosis of humans. We soon found that it was too high a dosage. We reduced it to five grams and later decided the correct dose was established at three grams."

There has not been a reported death from intravenous infusion of EDTA for twenty-five years. The dose given today is three grams for a usual number of one, two or maybe three treatments per week.

In support of Dr. Clarke, Dr. Halstead pointed out the significance of glomerulitis and nephritis mentioned in this 1954 case. This sort of support is needed currently even though you may find this talk about toxicity highly technical — even monotonous. Why is it needed? Because if you ask your traditional physician about whether or not you should take chelation therapy, he is going to quote you rumors he may have heard about this same 1954 case.

Dr. Halstead said, "It so happens that because of the work of Dow Chemical Company and others in producing versenate EDTA, which is used extensively for various food products, blood constituents, and other things, there have been very extensive studies in rats to determine whether or not there is any degree of renal [kidney] damage. In none of these reports have they ever reported glomerular nephritis. And if Dr. Clarke's case involves glomerular nephritis, we're talking about a patient complication — not EDTA toxicity. The fact that a person is being treated with EDTA and has atherosclerosis is no guarantee that he does not have pre-existing glomerular nephritis from other sources. He may have a host of other complications. Many of us don't just have arteriosclerosis. There are many other unknown entities.

"The dosage level is a very important point, too," said Dr. Halstead. "If the person was given five to ten grams of EDTA per day, he was far beyond the dosage range that is considered normal and accepted therapeutic dosage today."

Commenting on those first two deaths with EDTA therapy which were reported in the medical literature in 1955 and 1956, Garry F. Gordon, M.D.

of Sacramento, California suggested a comparison. Dr. Gordon, said, "The doses of EDTA used in those cases were 5 or 10 grams. You can compare this to an intake of water. Make the comparison! If you drank a year's supply of water in one week, you'd die, too. None the less, opponents of this therapy will continue to dwell on those singular cases, and any other negative stories they can twist to make it appear chelation is unsafe. They ignore the thousands of people who are treated successfully each year with no complications of any kind."

Findings on EDTA Safety by the Chelation Pioneer

Dr. Clarke, the chelation therapy pioneer, referring to EDTA safety, advised me, "Among the extensive publications verifying the therapeutic safety of EDTA is a work by Oser, Oser and Spencer, published in 1963,[17] that 'found EDTA generally considered to be quite innocuous.' In another study of theirs EDTA was fed in two times accepted strength for twelve weeks to weaning rats, 'it caused no signs of body injury,' they wrote."

Dr. Clarke also said, "Doolan and Schwartz of the United States Naval Medical Research Institute in 1967[14-16] studied the effect of EDTA on the kidneys and reported 'the label of nephrotoxicity (for EDTA) is unjustified.'

"Meltzer and Kitchell of the Hahnemann Medical School," Dr. Clarke continued, "published a report based on 2000 consecutive infusions of 3.0 gm. of EDTA and 'found *no* serious side effects or *toxicity* from EDTA when administered in 3.0 gm. doses — can be used over prolonged periods without evidence of toxicity.'[18]

"An unusual study on rotifers by Sincock was published in 1975 in the *Journal of Gerontology*. Sincock found 'significant increase in [rotifer] body calcium content with aging' and 'regular brief immersion periods [of rotifers] in a solution of EDTA with withdrawal of body calcium by chelation produced extension of life span and reproduction period'." *Rotifers* are a form of many-celled aquatic microorganisms having rows of cilia at one end, which in motion resemble revolving wheels. The rotifers were treated every other day of their lives with EDTA and lived 50 percent longer than controls.[19]

Dr. Clarke concluded, "From these and similar reports of which there are many, and from my own years spent in observing the therapeutic results and possible toxic effects of EDTA therapy and extensive clinical studies undertaken and published in 1955 and 1956, I conclude that EDTA deserves a place in the armament of the medical profession, even if it could help no more people than does our lauded present cancer therapy."

Relative Safety and LD-50 of EDTA

Dr. Bruce Halstead discussed any possible toxicity of EDTA with the California Medical Association's review committee on chelation therapy when he appeared at its March, 1976 hearing. Dr. Halstead said, "A great many statements have been made by a number of different organizations regarding the great hazard in the toxicity, the so-called nephrotoxicity of EDTA. In the field of toxicity we usually evaluate the toxicity of a substance based on its *LD-50*. We talk about a measure where the toxic ingredient produces death in about 50 percent of the organisms."

In explanation of Dr. Halstead's statement, I'll inform you about toxicity and *LD-50*. You must have two particular values to discuss intelligently toxicity of any drug. One value is the optimum effective dose and the other is the toxic dose of LD-50. *This LD-50 is the dose which, given over a specified period of time, will kill half the subjects the drug is being administered to*. The toxic dose divided by the therapeutic dose is the *therapeutic index*. This therapeutic index tells researchers and physicians how dangerous is a drug or other substance to living organisms, especially people.

If the therapeutic index is small, the compound or drug is toxic; if it is large, it is nontoxic. For example, if 1.0 gram per day is the optimum dose of a drug and 2.0 grams per day is the LD-50, the therapeutic index is two. Obviously this would be a very dangerous drug because the therapeutic index is small. Insulin may fall into this dangerous class. It has a low therapeutic index, and users know that insulin has to be administered with great caution. EDTA has an exceedingly high therapeutic index and is safer even than aspirin.

Dr. Halstead explained, "The LD-50 of EDTA is approximately 2,000 milligrams per kilogram of body weight, based on oral repetitive studies. And these studies have now been exhaustive and enormous. We find that the toxicity of EDTA can be compared to something we already are familiar with. That is the toxicity of aspirin. Aspirin's toxicity is 558 milligrams per kilogram of a person's body weight. So essentially, EDTA is about three and a half times *less* toxic than aspirin."

You can understand, therefore, that by Dr. Halstead's definition of EDTA toxicity this synthetic amino acid is less than one-third as toxic as aspirin. Aspirin is legally used as the treatment of headache, but EDTA has a much more important use. It improves blood flow to the heart, the head and the limbs.

Dr. Halstead's statement on the safety and non-toxicity of EDTA chelation therapy was confirmed in previous published reports.[18,20] EDTA has a wide safety spread of ten to 120 times between the therapeutic recommended dose and the LD-50. The recognition of depletion of trace minerals such as magnesium, zinc, chromium, manganese, and iron[20,21,22] and vitamin B depletion with appropriate replacement[23] has markedly improved its safety toward the high end of the scale. Even *teratogenesis*, the disturbed growth processes involved in the production of a malformed fetus, once reported in animals, was completely prevented with the administration of zinc.[24] Thus with an understanding of the mechanism of its action, the safety of EDTA, when given in recommended doses, seems firmly established.[18,25]

Chapter Eight

The Cost for Chelation Therapy

There is no greater reward in our profession than the knowledge that God has entrusted us with the physical care of His people. The Almighty has reserved for Himself the power to create life but He has assigned to a few of us the responsibility of keeping in good repair their bodies in which this life is sustained.
— Elmer Hess, M.D. past president, AMA.
American Weekly, April 24, 1955

Chelating Physicians Treat Their Own Loved Ones

For physicians who are exposed to the tragedies of illness, deterioration, and death caused by hardening of the arteries, no cost is too great to provide significant improvement in unhealthy lifestyles. Certain chelating physicians have encouraged, advised, pleaded, persuaded, and frightened their own loved ones into taking chelation treatment. They well know the benefits of this protection against the stress factors that are so pervasive in our polluted environment.

Robert B. Vance, D.O. of Salt Lake City, Utah is one such osteopathic physician who has undertaken protection of his family members and himself. I interviewed Dr. Vance by telephone, letter and in person.

"One of the reasons I use chelation therapy is that atherosclerotic disease runs in my family," Dr. Vance said. "My mother passed away from severe coronary atherosclerosis when she was sixty-eight years old. She had her first coronary at age fifty-eight. I watched her get progressively more restricted in movement. More and more she became limited and not responsive to conservative medical therapy. If only I had known about chelation therapy then. If only I was made aware of the use of chelation treatment in the United States and the work of Dr. Clarke of Birmingham, Michigan. If only information about the treatment had not been suppressed by the ingrained resistance to change of the medical establishment. The American medical profession's inability to accept something new like chelation has produced an apparent subtle conspiracy against the therapy. If only I had been able to use the treatment for my mother, I am sure she would be alive today.

"Now I've treated my father," continued Dr. Vance. "He is seventy-three years old, and he runs around like he is fifty-three. His main symptoms had been intermittent claudication [pain in the legs] when he climbed stairs and did other activities. He had ankle edema [swelling] and pain in the knees, too. I gave him twenty treatments two years ago and ten more this past summer [1976]. My father has no symptoms at all anymore. He takes no standard medication. He is on a full holistic program — nutritional and other therapeutic aides. He takes nothing of synthetic medicine — no drugs. He is doing just beautifully."

Dr. Vance has treated quite a number of his relatives with chelation therapy, including his wife and himself.

"Right now I am treating my uncle from Los Angeles," Dr. Vance said. "He is seventy-four years old and had suffered two near-fatal coronaries two-and-a-half and three years ago. On those two occasions he collapsed in his backyard. He described one of the attacks saying 'I thought my heart had exploded. This is it! This is the end!' Bam! He hit the deck but didn't die.

"I had been communicating with my uncle through family members for almost two years, encouraging him to come to Salt Lake City to get chela-tion," the physician said. "I am treating him now. He had been taking four different coronary medications, including nitroglycerine. After his third chelation treatment my uncle said, 'You know, Bob, I was able to sleep last night lying on my left side all night long without any pain in my chest. I haven't been able to do that for three years.' And after nine treatments my uncle no longer uses nitroglycerin. By September 1976, he took thirteen treatments, and he has started tapering off his other cardiac medication. I feel confident that he will go off all of his medication by the time we are finished with the full course of care."

Checking back with the osteopathic physician in June 1977, I learned that Dr. Vance's uncle is exceedingly well, after having taken twenty-five treat-ments. He has eliminated all of his prior cardiac medication. Now he main-tains himself with vitamins, minerals, regular exercise, and orthomolecular nutrition which includes the optimum diet against cardiovascular disease.

Chelating Physicians Take Treatment Themselves

In the March 1976 special meeting which looked at certain aspects of chelation therapy, Yiwen Y. Tang, M.D. of San Francisco told the ad hoc committee of the Scientific Advisory Board of the California Medical Associ-ation (CMA), "I was born in 1922. I have had thirty-eight treatments with chelation therapy — not in the expectation to cure any disease, but because I just wanted to do something preventic so that I may remain in the state of health I am now."

Bruce W. Halstead, M.D. of Loma Linda, California said to the same reviewing committee, "I'm sort of an asymptomatic junior in the business. I've received only thirteen treatments in terms of chelation therapy but plan to take a full twenty within the next few weeks." (My query to Dr. Halstead netted me more of his personal information in Feburary 1977. He said,

"Incidentally, I have now had twenty-four treatments.")

Garry F. Gordon, M.D. of Sacramento, California told the CMA, "I'm forty-one years old, and I've had approximately seventeen treatments. I was asymptomatic [had no health problems]. Using both plethysmography and thermography [with which to examine himself physically] before my treatments, my results were not to the 100 percent physiological ideal that I had decided to keep myself at. In spite of my being asymptomatic, I took chelation with EDTA. By the eighth treatment there were some interesting changes in myself that I observed. For instance, for the first time in my life I had the ability to stay at strenuous effort for an unlimited period of time, which previously I had not been able to do. This included running up a mountain."

And Charles H. Farr, M.D., Ph.D. of Norman, Oklahoma advised his colleagues, "I've had about thirty chelation treatments over the past two years. I've always been healthy, asymptomatic of any illness. I continue to be, and I hope I'll always be." To insure that his good health will remain, Dr. Farr told me in May 1977 that he took another series of chelations. And he has administered the treatment to every one of his relatives who consented to sit for it.

Dr. Farr Gave Both His Parents Chelation

Dr. Farr supplied for publication the case history and photographs of his mother, Mrs. W. E. (Myrtle) Farr of Oklahoma City, Oklahoma, who at the time of her arteriosclerotic problem was seventy-two years old. Myrtle Farr is a registered nurse, but she had discontinued working at her profession the previous year because of the onset of senility. Months were going by while she did nothing much more than live from day to day. Most days she could hardly drag herself from bed.

Dr. Farr said. "I was becoming concerned because my mother was confused, forgetful, and had lost all interest in life in general and herself in particular. She suffered with all the classical signs of *senile dementia*, or chronic brain syndrome, which is a result of cerebral arteriosclerosis. I started her on chelation therapy as soon as I could talk my father into taking the treatment, too. She refused to take it by herself.

"My mother was treated quite satisfactorily as you can see from the two photographs I have supplied. One picture was taken May 21, 1974 (see Photograph Ten) before I gave my mother chelation therapy. The other picture was taken August 29, 1974 (see Photograph Eleven) after she received a series of treatments. It indicates her change back to her former status as a very proud and alert person. In this later photograph she has become seventy-three years of age and returned to private duty nursing working full eight-hour shifts. The picture shows her wearing her nurse's uniform."

Dr. Farr said that, when dealing with cerebral arteriosclerosis, a chelating

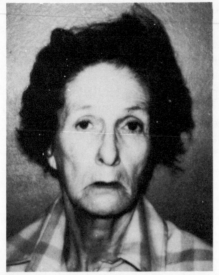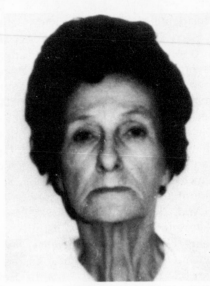

Mrs. Myrtle Farr was in an advanced state of senility in May 1974, when *Photograph 10* (left) was taken. Four months later, the 73-year-old nurse was able to return to her profession *(Photograph 11,* right), after a series of chelation treatments.

physician cannot predict the outcome of treatment. His own experience with administering EDTA infusion to approximately one hundred senile patients has shown him that significant improvement occurs in about 50 percent of these elderly people. He believes that a 50 percent chance of improvement is worth the investment of time and money in chelation therapy. His experience shows that while chelation is not a cure-all, it is far better than abandoning patients to a hopelessly impaired senile state.

In checking back with Dr. Farr in March 1979, I learned that Myrtle Farr, R.N. is still working and is able to outperform many other nurses who are much younger than she.

He added, "My father, W. E. Farr. who is seventy-seven years old, had arteriosclerotic heart disease before chelation therapy. Today he is living on a farm doing heavy manual labor and appears to be getting better and stronger with each day and week that goes by."

Dr. Harper Persuades His Mother

"After starting to practice chelation therapy," said Harold W. Harper, M.D. of Los Angeles, "I encouraged my mother for almost three years to take treatment from me. She was sixty-eight years old and had severe arthritis at the time. I saw the terrible condition she was in, limping and hardly able to walk. She was overweight and had high blood pressure. Finally her pain became so great she decided to try anything — even treatment from her son. When she arrived by plane for chelation she could not put one foot in front of the other without stumbling from stiffness and pain.

"I did a diagnostic workup on my mother and began the EDTA infusion. Between the fifth and seventh treatment she walked without a limp and had more energy than she'd shown in ten years. By the time she had taken the tenth treatment she was walking more than a mile a day and couldn't be held back because of her excess energy. There was no arthritic pain anymore and her blood pressure completely returned to normal," said Dr. Harper.

Physicians who employ chelation therapy for vascular occlusive conditions and other diseases find there is the return of a patient's function, in addition to relief of symptoms, as Dr. Harper had found. The rate of patient success is in the area of 80 percent.[1] Non-invasive tests easily remonitor improvement, and if regression has occurred, the patient's entire lifestyle can be reviewed and more chelation therapy given.

Alternately, if response to chelation has been inadequate and a surgical approach seems warranted, the patient will withstand surgery much better because of the EDTA intravenous injections. His general circulation has been improved by his having received the EDTA infusions. Even specific presenting conditions are often relieved by the nonspecific generalized chelation effects.

Invasive radiologic techniques, such as transluminal dilation[2,3] (the passage of light through dilated blood vessels), make chelation more efficacious by allowing better flow to the most obstructed areas. This will reduce the total number of chelation treatments required. There is no limitation as to who should be a recipient of the therapy. It is quite safe and almost riskless. Repeatedly angina symptoms have been relieved entirely even after the failure of two coronary bypass operations in the same patient.

The Financial Costs of Chelation Therapy

The cash required to finance chelation therapy varies around the country from a low of $50 per treatment to a high of $95. On the West Coast of the United States it tends toward the higher range. The fee along the Eastern seaboard averages about $75 per treatment. Some of these "price" differences relate not so much to the actual chelation infusion but to the adjunctive measures that are employed as well. Each treatment, for instance, may require you to take megadoses of vitamins and minerals because your body is deficient in these nutrients. The costs quoted sometimes include these adjunctive measures.

All the chelating physicians invariably request hair, urine, and/or saliva and feces tests in order to determine vitamin and mineral deficiencies. They do a diet analysis, too, so that you may receive the correct orthomolecular nutrition program specific for your need. The diet analysis forms are among the most thorough investigatory questionnaires I have ever seen. Results are returned to you from a computer. The computer printout tells you what food deficiencies you have and how you may alter your nutritional lifestyle.

Twenty chelation treatments is a usual series. However, twenty treatments are considered the *minimum course* for altering artery pathology that is *mild*. If given for medical *prevention* rather than as a corrective therapy, the number of infusions administered in a series may be less. Certainly twenty treatments is not enough to *reverse* a condition of hardening of the arteries that is *severe*, but the series can produce markedly improved functional changes throughout the circulatory system. Most persons' hearts do function better with a series of twenty EDTA infusions taken over seven to fourteen weeks. For the more severe occlusive arterial problems, probably thirty or forty treatments will be recommended for a single series of chelations. With various tests and examinations included, that initial total cost is likely to approach $2,000.

The Time Costs of Chelation Therapy

Among the larger problems faced by people who want EDTA chelation for preventive or therapeutic purposes is the expenditure of time. Cost alone is not the whole obstacle. An individual will ask himself, "How can I visit the doctor's office twice a week and remain there for four to six hours each visit? Can I afford the time? Won't I lose money? Who will run my business? How can I explain it to my boss?"

Most physicians find it difficult to get people to invest time in themselves. The motivation must come from within the individual. A person has to reorder his priorities if preventive medicine and prolonged life is part of one's major desires.

On the other hand, heart pain that strikes an individual cannot be argued with. Days, weeks, and months will be found for bed confinement to recuperate from a heart attack. If circulatory distress has turned a leg gangrenous, somehow a person finds the time to have the amputation that will save his life.

"I was no different," said Warren M. Levin, M.D. of New York City. "I decided I was going to take chelation several years ago, and I just never got around to it because I thought I couldn't afford the time. Finally I told myself that I've just got to do it! I managed to arrange for the therapy at the end of my full working day. I ate dinner, relaxed a little, then got into bed, put the needle into my own vein, and went to sleep. A registered nurse, whom I had hired at regular nursing rates, sat by my bedside all night for a full-eight-hour shift to keep the intravenous drip going at the correct speed. She made sure the chelate did not infiltrate into surrounding tissues. The financial cost to me actually was greater than it is to one of my patients. I was paying a nurse's wages for all those hours that I slept."

Individual treatment times vary for patients, but on the average EDTA administration takes four to five hours. It will be shorter — as little as two and a half hours — if the patient can tolerate a faster drip. It will be longer —

as long as eight hours — if the patient has a sensitivity reaction to the components in the EDTA solution.

From one to three treatments per week is a usual number, two per week being most common. This will be the schedule except in those instances where the patient has traveled far for a short stay in a hospital facility or doctor's clinic. Then treatment will be given for five days in a row with a two-day pause and five days consecutively again. This consecutive treatment also is administered when the patient is in danger of imminent death and radical measures are required. This daily frequency has been safely applied to thousands of people for over twenty years. The thinking by chelating physicians is changing, however. Current medical malpractice conditions and other legal considerations are causing many physicians today to opt for the ultraconservative program of one, two, or maybe three treatments per week. As more doctors adopt chelation in more cities, it may someday be possible to avoid lodging and meal costs altogether.

The Cost in Skill and Training

The actual technique of chelation administration does not take much skill on the part of medical professionals. Almost anyone can give it — like delivering a baby — even paraprofessionals perform the technique well. That is one of the aspects of this treatment that upsets organized medicine; no extra special training is required. Any physician anywhere can give it to his patient. Medical service monopoly is taken from the hands of super specialists, such as cardiologists, internists, vascular surgeons, chest surgeons, anesthesiologists, and various maintainers of sophisticated hospital facilities. The rendering of medical services is handed back to the general practitioner when he or she administers chelation therapy.

The generally trained medical practitioner or his nurse can take on the responsibility of administration, and that is the key here — *responsibility*. A medical professional has to be able to responsibly react to the patient's possible discomfort during administration or to any side effects afterward. This means simply that the doctor should be knowledgeable in the technique. He or she must attend medical meetings oriented to chelation therapy. He or she also might tour the facilities of other chelating physicians and, of course, the doctor who chelates has to do a *lot* of reading on the subject.

Then you might wonder why, if the treatment is so easy and so simple to administer, the cash costs should be relatively high. There are several pertinent reasons to explain the charges.

First, you must be in the doctor's office for so many hours. During that time the doctor and his staff are responsible for your well-being. Patients pay the physician to take that responsibility.

Second, chelation physicians usually require larger offices and more employees to accommodate the huge amount of traffic that moves in and out. This results in significantly larger overhead to pay.

Next, the physician who chelates must take the time from his practice for attendance at the required expensive conventions.

Finally, the chelating physician usually has to retain several competent attorneys. Why? Because patients, you and I, have to pay for the doctor's legal risk and the peer pressure he gets from organized medicine. Several chapters that follow tell of the politics involved with chelation therapy. You will read of the intra- and interprofessional stress physicians must face for daring to offer EDTA chelation to their patients.

The Cost of a Singular Chelation Case

Illustrative of the costs in time, money, and anxiety connected with chelation therapy is the singular case of George Kavic of West Mifflin, Pennsylvania. He is a retired foreman on permanent disability from United States Steel Corporation. Living on a pension as he does, Kavic did not have the "cash on the barrelhead" required for extensive chelation therapy. Nor did he have the time to earn the cash by taking odd jobs, because he was told by his doctors, "George, don't make any definite plans. You have only three to six months to live!"

Kavic suffered constant pains and burning sensations because three-fourths of his myocardium had been damaged by a series of heart attacks. The angina he felt was so great it took him five minutes to move just ten yards across a room. Additionally, his right leg was so circulatorily deficient, it turned blue and claudicated with any weight bearing. His doctors said that they hoped the leg would not have to be amputated because the patient would never survive the operation.

During our 1977 interview, George Kavic said, "In November 1975 my cardiologist told me the results of my angiogram. He said that bypass surgery wasn't possible even though I needed it in both my leg and my chest. I had blockage of two coronary arteries that narrowed their openings by 80 percent and 90 percent. The risk that I would die on the operating table was too great.

"I asked the cardiologist what he thought about my taking chelation therapy, and he said that I was nuts to consider it! He said also, 'If you are still living in September (1976) then make an appointment with me for that following December. You may make it that long, but you have a very tough case.' So I was left waiting to die, but while waiting I had terrible and unbearable pain in my right leg," Kavic said. "I didn't tell my wife because it would frighten her to death. It was blue up to the ankle, and I couldn't walk at all."

Out of desperation, and over his cardiologist's objections, the patient telephoned Dr. Evers to inquire about the chelation treatment. Learning the therapy's cost, Kavic knew that such funds were out of his grasp. But he knew, too, that no alternative lay open whereas chelation therapy did offer some possibility of relieving his condition at least a little. He hoped he could squeeze another year of life out of having the treatment. Therefore, George Kavic borrowed $6,500 from loving friends and relatives. He knew from Dr. Ever's telephone estimate that about thirty chelations were required to be given daily with a pause on the weekends. That would be five or six weeks of hospitalization that he had to finance, besides the airfare south to the hospital where Dr. Evers administered the treatment.

The trip south had Kavic almost exhausted. He experienced feelings of tremendous anxiety. "I was scared," Kavic confessed. "I wondered if this trip was worth it."

The patient took thirty-two chelation treatments in November 1975. Physical improvement began for him at about the fourth treatment day. After one week he telephoned home to report that he was able to walk a mile without feeling chest pains or leg pains. After five weeks Kavic's pedometer showed that he walked six miles a day without any difficulty.

George Kavic told me, "I haven't had the return of symptoms. I have no family doctor anymore. I don't take any medication, except with each meal I add five food supplements that I buy at a health food store. I swallow these vitamins with my food, and I feel like a million dollars. I walk regularly four, five, and six miles a day because that's part of my rehabilitation program — regular exercise. I returned for a recheck of my laboratory tests about ten months after the chelation treatment. The readouts were magnificent. Dr. Evers showed me that my triglycerides, cholesterol and other tests all showed improvement over the first time. Then I had five more bottles of the EDTA solution too, for a total of thirty-seven treatments."

At this writing George Kavic looks like a classic example of good health. He is energetic and forceful — so much so that occasionally he pushes himself to the point of heart pain. Those pains remind him that once he was told he had less than six months to live.

Chapter Nine

Health Insurance Coverage for Intravenous Chelation Therapy

The private insurance companies have been a massive success in selling health insurance, but they have been an equally massive failure in providing cost control and effective health coverage. The companies are so preoccupied with writing up new policies that they have written off any responsibility for the health system. The insurance industry works for profit. To the insurance companies, people are the enemy, because every private claim is a threat to corporate profit.
— U.S. Senator Edward M. Kennedy, *The American Legion Magazine,* July, 1971

The Cure of Mr. Aubrey Is Not Usual and Customary

Alfred Aubrey of San Diego, California is sixty-eight years old and an eligible Medicare recipient. He appreciates the Social Security benefits he receives when he gets them. Mr. Aubrey was recently relieved of the symptoms of coronary artery heart disease. He was saved from having another heart attack, too. But since the treatment this Medicare recipient received was something other than open heart surgery, the Social Security Administration refused to pay his doctor's bill.

"Regardless of the desperateness of Mr. Aubrey's health situation, and regardless of the effectiveness of the treatment, there is no coverage," ruled the Medicare hearing officer. The Federal Government in effect decided how the patient could be treated and how he could use his body. Why? Why should the Medicare insurance carrier and the government's hearing officer deny payment for chelation therapy to save a life? Because "this was not the *usual and customary* treatment for the conditions diagnosed," said Clyde H. Burgardt, the hearing officer.

Alfred Aubrey received intravenous chelation therapy for angina pains, diabetes, and post-cardiovascular accident. He had been suffering from acute atherosclerosis of the coronary arteries and was in immediate danger of being struck down by a second heart attack. Nevertheless, the involved insurance carrier for Medicare, Occidental Life Insurance Company of California, which was obligated to pay eighty percent of the patient's $515 medical bill, reimbursed him only $8.50 — even though he is a worthy

Medicare recipient. Sounds silly — downright ridiculous — doesn't it? Shrugging your shoulders you might say, "Well I don't know Medicare's side of the story." OK! I'll lay out the facts, and you be the judge.

The following information comes directly from Hearing Officer Burgardt's decision document, dated September 10, 1976. Mr. Burgardt is an independent licensed insurance claim adjuster of San Gabriel, California. He was called upon to conduct a "Fair Hearing" in San Diego to decide on benefits the insurance recipient deserved under Part B of the Medicare Program.

A Brief Explanation of Medicare

Medicare is a program of medical insurance under the Social Security Act passed into law in 1965. The program offers people over age sixty-five health insurance and consists of two parts.

Part A, *hospital insurance*, is basic, and is financed out of compulsory contributions paid by employers and workers in their working years. It tends to be more liberally administered in that it pays for therapies that are not "usual and customary."

Part B, *medical insurance*, is supplementary and optional. It helps to pay "allowable charges" for doctors' and surgeons' fees and other medical services and items not included under hospital insurance. Persons over age sixty-five voluntarily pay a monthly premium of $8.70 for Part B, and the Federal Government matches the sum. Also the participant pays the first $60 of expenses for covered services in a calendar year and twenty percent of the annual costs above $60.

Unlike the hospitals who are direct payment recipients, claimants of Part B must request their own reimbursements by filling out forms and sending them to the appropriate insurance carrier office. The claimants may offer assignment of benefits to servicing doctors if the doctors will accept them. Otherwise, claimants must pay the medical bills and attempt to get reimbursed from the carrier.

Part B medical insurance covers: (1) Physicians' and surgeons' services; (2) home health services ordered by a doctor up to 100 visits a year, even if the patient has not been in a hospital; (3) other health and medical equipment, surgical dressings and splints, and diagnostic tests. [1, 2]

Millions of Part B Medicare dollars are spent annually by health insurance carriers. The insurance companies are paid administrative fees to spend participants' and U.S. taxpayers' money (channeled through the Social Security Administration). Every payment request usually is subjected to rigid scrutiny under insurance regulations over which we, the medical consumers, have no control. Because insurance home office people seem to assume in advance that all claims are fraudulent or excessive, the claimant is treated as if he is a crook. This is the usual insurance company practice, as the quote by Senator Edward Kennedy, which I used to open this chapter, says: "To the insurance companies, people are the enemy . . ." If health insurance companies can "save" money for Uncle Sam's health programs, more of the funds may become available for "administrative purposes" — that is, home office wages, salary increases and bonuses. Wherever the insurance company employees can, they "save."

The Shocking Case of Alfred Aubrey

Alfred Aubrey is a Medicare Part B participant and early in 1975, for the second time in his life, his heart was seized with pain. The angina was so knife-like he was unable to perform any substantial physical activity. He could not even carry on as a church usher. The slightest exertion — including slow walking — brought on severe chest pains. A surgeon to whom he went for help advised Mr. Aubrey that he was in dire danger of death. His need, he was told, was to have open heart surgery for correction of his angina. But the heart surgeon warned also that the mortality risk for him in such a surgery was fifty percent. He had a 50-50 chance of dying from the operation.

Despite the threat of death, the patient consented to the operation anyway. Subsequent hospital tests then showed Mr. Aubrey was not eligible — not a fit candidate — for open heart surgery. In effect, he was refused the operation and left to die.

The hopeless man turned to William J. Saccoman, M.D. of San Diego, California, who is a specialist in family practice and psychiatry. The patient appealed to Dr. Saccoman for any possible solution to his several health problems. Mr. Aubrey left it to the physician to choose the type of treatment, and he paid for the various services that were rendered.

After receiving a course of chelation care from Dr. Saccoman during the period March 3, 1975 to April 25, 1975, the patient's chest pains disappeared. Clyde Burgardt wrote: "He was able to resume normal physical activities, without bringing on a return of the angina," a direct quote from the Fair Hearing officer's record. "His blood pressure returned to well within normal limits, and his heart action has been good subsequent to and as a result of the services performed by Dr. Saccoman," Mr. Burgardt continued.

Aubrey testified at the Medicare Fair Hearing that now he walks four miles daily, before breakfast, and this he was able to do shortly after being treated with EDTA chelation. Also his blood sugar level, which had been elevated from diabetes, returned to normal.

In June 1975, Aubrey, now a *former* heart victim, visited another physician, Dr. Cooper. The patient went strictly for his personal gratification in order to get a medical checkup by an impartial observer. Dr. Cooper pronounced the man's heart good and his lungs clear. He could no longer be considered a cardiac patient.

Was it reasonable and necessary for Alfred Aubrey to seek help from Dr. Saccoman? Is it something you would have done to save your own life? Do you believe Medicare, Part B should have compensated this retired person for payment of the physician's bill in the amount of $364.00, which is the amount arrived at after the patient pays $60 and twenty percent of the balance? The sum due for reimbursement consists of eighty percent of the bill for which the carrier was responsible, but the carrier paid only $8.50.

Regulation 405.310, as set forth in the Hearing Officers Handbook, states that Medicare, Part B, shall make no payment for services "which are not reasonable and necessary for the diagnosis or treatment of illness or injury. . . ." Occidental Life Insurance Company of California disallowed the expense of Aubrey's chelation therapy. The carrier had labeled the treatment "experimental and not tested, as to treatment of arteriosclerotic heart disease" and "is not considered the usual and customary treatment."

The hearing officer ruled only on the question of what was "reasonable and necessary." The decision he rendered said, "The controlling thing here is that the Law, Regulations and Guidelines do provide coverage *only* for usual and customary treatment for the conditions diagnosed. The greater weight of evidence here is that this treatment was not the usual and customary treatment for the conditions diagnosed. Therefore, regardless of the desperateness of Mr. Aubrey's health situation, and regardless of the effectiveness of the treatment, there is no coverage."

If the patient had been accepted as a candidate for open heart surgery, Occidental Life Insurance Company of California, representing Medicare, Parts B and A, would have paid the whole $15,000 coronary bypass surgical fee, plus the accompanying hospital costs — about $10,000 more, less the small amount for which the patient was responsible. And with that $25,000 expenditure, Mr. Aubrey was told his chance of *survival* was only fifty percent! Nevertheless, the carrier refused to reimburse for chemical endarterectomy with EDTA, a safe and life-preserving procedure. And its refusal was upheld by this "Fair Hearing."

Following such a "Fair Hearing," elderly citizens supposedly covered by Part B Medicare, but denied the benefits owed them, are informed that they have *no* recourse to the courts — and they do not! There is no appeal from the hearing officer's decision.

Medicare, Part B Also Refuses Payment for Pre-Chelation Tests

It has been reported that twenty percent of vein grafts put in place as substitutes for occluded portions of coronary arteries become occluded themselves within one year of surgery. Vein grafts, in fact, have been shown as accelerators of disease in the very same arteries that receive the grafts. A new total occlusion occurs not infrequently on either side of the graft.[3,6]

New occlusions *did* take place in the arteries of Walter W. Watson of San Francisco after he had been subjected to two previous heart attacks and had undergone two bypass operations, performed one after the other in September 1972. Both heart surgeries were covered by medical and hospital insurance to the tune of $25,000 per procedure. The reoccurrence of occlusions of his coronary arteries affected Mr. Watson in the fall of 1974. The slightest physical effort, even slow walking, caused him tremendous chest pain. A third heart operation seemed a certainty, but he was not anxious to face bypass surgery again.

Walter Watson brought his health problem to Garry F. Gordon, M.D., then the director of the Sacramento (California) Medical Preventics Clinic, who administered chelation therapy to him from November 14, 1974 through January 8, 1975. The patient realized great therapeutic benefit with complete elimination of his discomfort.

Watson paid his $1,393.75 bill to Dr. Gordon for medical services rendered and, since he was a Medicare beneficiary, submitted the bill for reimbursement to Blue Shield of California, the responsible Part B, Medicare carrier. But Blue Shield of California allowed only $10.00 of the total billed. It was an allowance for just one office visit. Payment for the remainder of the services was refused on the grounds that the Social Security Administration has specifically stated that the services and tests connected with chelation therapy are not a benefit of the Medicare program.

A Fair Hearing was requested by the Sacramento Medical Preventics Clinic on behalf of Mr. Watson. The hearing was held in the Sacramento, California Social Security Administration office on August 25, 1976.

In attendance at the hearing were Dr. Gordon, Robert Wolfe, M.D., who is a Blue Shield of California medical advisor, and Elizabeth Rossi, an administrative representative of the carrier. C. W. Lemming of San Francisco was the Medicare hearing officer. I have in my possession the tape-recorded transcript of that meeting.

Mrs. Rossi quoted from the Medicare Carriers' Manual, Part 3, Section 2050.4(D)(1)(b) which states, "Endrate (EDTA) may be considered a benefit of the Medicare program only for the emergency treatment of hypercalcemia, and or control of ventricular arrhythmias and heart block associated with digitalis toxicity." Walter Watson was *not* a victim of these conditions.

Dr. Wolfe said, "Chelation is not a benefit, and when a service is not a benefit the tests done to monitor it, such as in this case: the quantitative urines, the biofeedback, the thermography (and the plethysmography), also are deleted. These tests are not payable. This is a specific regulation. Now we could discuss this matter until doomsday, but it is not in our jurisdiction. This is up to the Bureau of Health Insurance and the FDA [Food and Drug Administration] to make the decision. When they have it they will put it down in [Medicare] regulations and then we can pay it. Until then our hands are tied."

Dr. Gordon asked, "Would you agree that if I did an electrocardiogram [EKG], and it comes back showing ischemic heart disease then my judgement must have been correct to have done the procedure?"

Dr. Wolfe replied, "An EKG is payable as part of the standard physical examination on a patient with cardiac symptoms."

Dr. Gordon said, "OK! Then a patient who has symptoms of vascular disease and is unable to walk [such as Mr. Watson] and has loss of memory, central nervous system symptoms, probably carotid artery disease, and whose study comes back positive, would have to be paid because it is obvious that an EKG is no more accepted a procedure then plethysmography or thermography (when performed prior to chelation therapy)."

Dr. Wolfe said, "This, again, is beyond our jurisdiction because the level of the screening test is something that regulations dictate and not us."

Dr. Gordon said, "Dr. Wolfe, are you going to state that this man, who came to me unable to walk, with two previous heart attacks, is being *screened* for arteriosclerosis when I do these tests on him?"

Dr. Wolfe answered meekly, "No, I'm not."

Dr. Gordon said, "Then let's get that clear! I have checked with Cedars of Lebanon Hospital in Los Angeles prior to coming to this meeting. Hal Ross, D.Sc., of the hospital's Non-invasive Vascular Laboratory advised me that they charge exactly twice what I charge for plethysmography and thermography, and they get paid for outpatient care by Southern California Medicare every single day. Just because my physician reviewer [who is the same Dr. Wolfe in Northern California] is not knowledgeable about these areas [diagnostic techniques] doesn't mean it is not accepted by medical experts around the country such as at Harvard University Medical School and the University of Vermont Medical Center."

Dr. Wolfe and Mrs. Rossi then admitted that they specifically do not make Medicare payments for diagnostic tests to determine the feasibility of using *chelation therapy* on a patient because chelation therapy is considered "investigational" and "experimental."

Once again the specter of closed minds among Medicare bureaucrats was causing these people to deny reimbursement even for diagnostic tests connected with heart disease prior to chelation. Yet, every reputable journal that physicians read regarding *bypass surgery* says it remains an investigational and essentially experimental procedure. Famous heart surgeon Denton Cooley told a medical convention that the surgical bypass procedure will probably be stopped in 1980. But Medicare, Part A and B, do pay all costs less usual deductibles for the bypass operation.

Still, in the opinion of Mr. Lemming, the Fair Hearing Officer, the clinical and laboratory tests and treatments received by Walter W. Watson were not considered a benefit of the Medicare program. The patient was refused reimbursement of his medical bill, even for the diagnostic tests.

The irony and injustice of this ruling against Mr. Watson is that the diagnostic tests were performed to measure accurately the extent of his vascular disease. These same test costs would have been paid if they had been performed by any other facility besides a clinic where chelation therapy is carried out. This is true by Medicare's own rulings. The tests should have been paid when done by Dr. Gordon's clinic. But organized medicine today steadfastly refuses to recognize the value of chelation, possibly because they don't really understand it. And organized medicine in large measure determines what health insurance benefits will and will not be paid.

A Private Group Health Insurance Carrier Will Not Cover Chelation

Typical of this sort of violation of a patient's health insurance rights was another non-payment ruling after the patient applied to a private group health insurance carrier to fulfill contract obligations for which the policy holder paid premiums. The violation was experienced by John Michaels of Woodenville, Washington.

At age forty-five, Mr. Michaels developed disabling angina pectoris. His visit to a cardiologist for an exercise tolerance test with electrocardiogram showed that he was the victim of severe ischemia of the heart muscle. He suffered with two millimeters of S-T segment depression on his electrocardiogram. This degree of depression indicates an impaired coronary blood flow.

Mr. Michaels was stunned by the realization that he was now unable to fulfill his long-time dream to become a gentleman farmer. The farm he had just purchased was useless to him. He could not pick up a spade-load of dirt without being incapacitated by angina pain. His cardiologist recommended the coronary bypass operation as the *only* option available. Michaels wasn't convinced, however, and he pondered his decision.

Another doctor, Leo J. Bolles, M.D. of Bellevue, Washington, had been the Michaels' family physician for a while. "John Michaels came to visit me to discuss whether or not he should have the coronary bypass surgery done," said Dr. Bolles. "I pointed out that there really was an alternative, and the patient elected not to have the operation performed but to try chelation therapy first.

"I administered ten chelation treatments to him," Dr. Bolles said. "I then cautiously performed a two-step electrocardiograph which turned out to be positive, although it was not as bad as had been his previous readings.

"I administered another ten chelations to the patient and exercised him again on a two-step test. He was still slightly positive but by this time had absolutely no anginal pain symptoms. He could work seven hours a day doing hard manual labor on his farm.

"I gave him a third series of ten chelations and then decided to send Mr. Michaels back to the cardiologist to have a new cardiological evaluation."

With a smile Dr. Bolles said, "This cardiologist exercised him very vigorously for about five minutes. He walked the patient up and down the two-step for the whole time, but the doctor could not produce any symptoms of coronary ischemia. Mr. Michaels no longer showed any S-T segment depression on his electrocardiograph. The cardiologist sent me a copy of the tracing but didn't interpret it. And the patient has been asymptomatic since."

Although at the outset of treatment Michaels had been told by Dr. Bolles that health insurance refuses to pay for chelation therapy, the recovered patient submitted a claim anyway. His logic was that if he had acceded to the orthodox medical option — heart surgery (which is clearly experimental and unproven) — his private policy would have paid the bills without a murmur. The same health insurance should then cover the tests and treatment he did choose, Michaels reasoned. But it did not.

The Prudential Life Insurance Company was the private carrier for group health insurance issued by the Teamsters' Union in Seattle. Michaels was a holder of that union's insurance plan. For this heart patient that private carrier was, literally, making a decision for John Michaels of how he must treat his body. The insurance company was determining his treatment for him, according to the dictates of its policy clauses and by its payment or non-payment of his health-connected bills.

Michaels and Correll Confront the Health Insurance Carrier

Michaels became angry when the reply to his claim stated that the therapy he had selected was not "usual and necessary." "Usual, chelation treatment may not be," the patient said, "but *necessary* for me, it sure as hell was!"

He went directly to the insurance company offices to demand a hearing. Surprising as it may sound, the hearing was not granted until two years later. William D. Correll, who is Dr. Bolles' business manager, accompanied the patient at this time and attended a two-hour meeting with Prudential Insurance Company representatives. Mr. Correll also is Executive Director of the Northwestern Academy of Preventive Medicine.

"I sat down at the table with the chief Prudential representative," said William Correll in a 1979 interview with me. "He opened a folder and stated, 'We are following chelation very closely across the country.' "

Correll replied, "Let's get to the facts in the case at hand. Mr. Michaels was suffering angina. He could not work at all. He suffered with intermittent claudication and a host of other health problems. Today his condition is altogether improved. He's working eight hours a day plus running this large farm. He has no angina. The pain left him during the course of treatment and has not returned to this point which is two years afterward. The patient is well. Those are the facts!"

At that meeting, Michaels and Correll met with narrow minds and rule book regulations as if they had struck against a stone wall. The stock insurance industry phrase, "this is not usual and customary procedure," was heard over and over.

Correll said, "That insurance representative told me, 'It really doesn't matter to us whether the patient got well or died. What matters to us is that the doctor did not use usual and customary procedure.' For John Michaels, what was usual and customary might possibly have killed him," concluded William Correll.

Medicare, Part A Is Forced to Pay for Chelation Care

If both kinds of carriers, the private health insurance companies and the carriers that administer Medicare, Part B, deny reimbursement to policy holders who take chelation care, is any chelation insurance available? Yes, Medicare, Part A, the hospital protection for U.S. citizens sixty-five years old and older, provides reimbursement for payment of therapeutic EDTA chelation bills. The payment will be made if service is rendered in a hospital. Medicare, Part A, has been forced by legal precedent to pay hospitals for the costs involved with chelation. Be advised, however, that each case is judged individually.

The precedent was set in the case of Mr. D. D. Dominey, Sr., of Atlanta, Georgia who was sixty-nine years old at the time of his admission to Columbia General Hospital, Andalusia, Alabama, from November 29, to December 11, 1970. That was the practice location of H. Ray Evers, M.D. before he moved to Montgomery, Alabama.

Mr. Dominey had been the head of three corporations, but then he found himself becoming senile and unable to function. He withdrew as corporate chief.

Dominey had a fifteen-year history of heart and angina attacks and had suffered a cerebral vascular accident (stroke) with some apparent hemorrhage into the cerebral tissue. He was experiencing numbness in his right arm and hand, a cough and chest pain upon exertion, severe pain in his legs at night, weakness, anxiety, tension, and severe precordial pain. Despite his medications, which were nitroglycerine and cardilate, his condition was becoming worse. His ophthalmologist testified that after he had examined Dominey's eyes and had seen the terrible condition of his blood vessels, he advised the patient to be hospitalized or his health problem could be fatal.

Upon the patient's admission to Columbia General Hospital, H. Ray Evers, M.D. administered extensive diagnostic tests to him. The result was a diagnosis of coronary heart disease, arteriosclerotic heart disease, and moderately severe generalized arteriosclerosis. Dr. Evers decided on chelation therapy as the method of treatment. Dominey received ten intravenous infusions of Endrate®, daily myoflex treatments (a form of physical therapy), medications, and a special diet. His condition was closely monitored to make certain that any essential minerals lost during chelation were replaced. He improved steadily and was discharged greatly improved, although he was still feeling numbness in his arm and hand.

Chelation Therapy Makes Dominey a New Man

Within a few weeks of treatment Dominey found he was able to discontinue his cardilate and seldom had to take a nitroglycerine pill. The opthalmologist, upon a re-examination of the patient's eyes, was amazed to observe that he was like a new person after chelation therapy.

In fact, Dominey *felt* like a new person. His angina had gone away altogether and he could walk all he wanted. He was subject to absolutely no intermittent claudication, no night pain, no chest pain, and once again he found himself sexually potent where he had not been so before EDTA chelation. He got married. He again took over total control of the three corporations in which he held stock.

Dominey paid the hospital's $3,500 bill for the chelation therapy he had received, and then filed for Medicare, Part A reimbursement for which he was qualified. Medicare refused the reimbursement.

Having considerable independent wealth, and with a long history behind him of having paid large Federal taxes, and having made Social Security payments for himself and his employees, Mr. Dominey decided to demand the Medicare money to which he was entitled. He sued the Social Security Administration for hospital insurance benefits under Title XVIII of the Social Security Act, as amended.

Now you should be made aware of the unique system under which Social Security is administered. For instance, the Social Security System has its own court system. The legal administrators, judges, and hearing officers are all hired and paid salaries by the Social Security Administration. In other words, they are dependent for their paychecks upon a system that they are asked to rule for or against. They make rulings in areas where they have a conflict of interests which would likely favor their employer.

There is an arbitration level in the Social Security System to which a plaintiff applies before he sues. Dominey made application for arbitration and then won his case at that level. The System's arbitrator had ruled against the Social Security Administration, who was his own boss, since the facts spoke for themselves. The Dominey case was that strong.

However, the Social Security Administration did not accept the arbitrator's ruling. It had a lot to lose if it did. Just how much is at stake if Medicare must pay for chelation therapy, I shall disclose more fully in Chapter Twelve.

Dominey Wins Case After Case

The Dominey case progressed up the line with multiple appeals. The first appeal was heard October 12, 1973 by Judge Cutler, who also found for the claimant and ruled that Medicare should reimburse him. The Social Security Administration, realizing that this might set a precedent for payments to several thousand other patients, appealed the case to the next higher administrative Social Security Court.

Dominey's case did not come up again for about a year and a half. By that time Judge Cutler, who had heard the first appeal, had become a higher appeals court judge in the administrative law system. He reheard the appeal himself on February 24, 1975. Social Security Courts are not legal courts but are administrative only, and it was legitimate for the judge to reassess his own prior decision.

To collect $3,500 in paid medical expenses Dominey was spending up-wards of $15,000 in legal fees and other expenses. Medical experts flew to Atlanta, where the appeals hearings were held. Additional costs amounting to $10,000 were paid out by physician witnesses themselves in travel ex-penses, lost wages, and lost time. Expert witnesses included Drs. Bruce Halstead, H. Ray Evers, Harold W. Harper, Norman Clarke, Sr., and others. Dominey again won his case.

The Social Security Administration still refused to give in. It had all the U.S. taxpayer money it needed for legal costs, and tried for a last time to reverse the decision.

The Social Security Administration brought a motion for review to the Appeals Council in Atlanta, presided over by council members Marshall C. Gardner and Irwin Friedenberg. More money was spent for more witnesses to appear. Dominey persisted with his claim and dipped into his pocket again. Finally he won! The Appeals Council's opinion was that "the claim-ant's twelve-day hospital stay was *reasonable and necessary*." Dominey's win was a benefit for every Medicare, Part A recipient — within limitations.

Among other findings in Mr. Dominey's favor, the two Appeals Council members wrote: "It was *reasonable and necessary* that the extensive diagnostic testing be given the claimant on an in-patient basis because he was severe-ly ill.

"When chelation therapy was decided as the proper course of treatment, it was *reasonable and necessary* that these treatments be given the claimant on an in-patient basis so that his condition could be properly monitored.

"The Claimant received services which were *reasonable and necessary* to be given by professional medical personnel on an in-patient basis for treatment of his illnesses.

"It is the decision of the Appeals Council that payment may be made on the claimant's behalf under Part A of Title XVIII of the Social Security Act for the services furnished him by Columbia General Hospital from November 29 to December 11, 1970. The decision of the administration law judge is hereby affirmed."

The decision was handed down December 1, 1975 and Dominey collected his reimbursement soon after that. In that way, Medicare, Part A was forced to pay for chelation care, but it still fights each recipient's payment request on an individual basis.

The Health Insurance Conspiracy Against Us

It is obvious to anyone who reads the signs that the health insurance industry has conspired and is conspiring to avoid paying patients' claims wherever it can get away with it. Insurance carriers are in subtle conspiracy in part by their abrogation of our freedom of choice to select the therapy we require and the therapy our physicians recommend. Being of sound mind, having complete information, and feeling full confidence in our physicians, we are owed the right to seek various medical alternatives besides what the medical profession establishment dictates is "usual and customary" and what the health insurance industry decides is "necessary and reasonable."

Breach of contract is being perpetrated on every person who holds a health insurance policy. *"Premium Payer Be Damned"* is the overriding motto of health insurance industry leaders when it comes to chelation therapy. They use political agitation to intensify what best fits their own industrial health and not the public's physical and mental health. A strong insurance lobby in Washington attempts to supplant the law in taxation. It nets the insurance companies tax-free buildings and other tax-free properties. If they are able to alter the tax laws in their favor, isn't it logical that they would attempt the manipulation of therapies, too? They have made exactly that attempt and have been exceedingly successful.

The insurance industry, which is supposed to furnish underwriting guarantees and protection of the nation's health, is able to suppress therapy through local medical societies that are uninformed or misinformed. As a result, the *only* procedures they recommend just happen to be horribly expensive, require the services of many highly trained (and costly) specialists, involve lengthy hospital stays — and are only marginally successful!

Bypass surgery is among these silver pocket-lining procedures foisted on the unknowing American public by medical pressure groups (as we shall see in the next chapter). Another way organized medicine lines its pockets with health insurance company silver is with drug therapy for which health insurance policies pay. Drug therapy supports many medical functions, such as the publication of medical journals, the running of conventions, and other physician activities related to health. The physician members of organized medicine often carry investment portfolios filled with drug stocks and various business-health enterprises.

In fact, many practicing physicians in the medical mainstream sit on the boards of directors of these health-related enterprises. More often than not, they are the very physicians who influence health insurance company decisions. The health insurance industry responds to the medical care industry. They conspire jointly, as you are about to learn.

Chapter Ten
Bypass Surgery: The Controversial Antagonist to Chelation Therapy

Surgery is always second best. If you can do something else, it's better. Surgery is limited. It is operating on someone who has no place else to go.
— John Kirklin, M.D., heart surgeon,
Mayo Clinic, *Time*, May 3, 1963

Don't Get Chest Pains in Spokane

"Get chest pains in Spokane, Washington and ninety minutes later you'll be on the operating table with your sternum split open having a triple bypass," says Harold W. Harper, M.D. On a number of occasions, in interviews I recorded and from the public speaking platform before groups of holistic physicians, Dr. Harper has told the story of the marvelous efficiency of Spokane chest surgeons. The last time he described their skill was at the May 1979 semi-annual meeting of the American Academy of Medical Preventics held in Chicago. It's a tale that has you breathless and somewhat dismayed.

Public and private ambulance companies in Spokane speed any person complaining of chest pains to a particular hospital emergency room. As the ambulance dashes through crowded streets, the driver radios ahead, and the surgical team assembles in readiness. No time is wasted in case a cardiopulmonary bypass surgery is needed.

Bypass surgery is a shunting operation in which a vascular prosthesis is used between the aorta femoral artery to relieve obstruction of the lower abdominal aorta, its bifurcation, and the proximal iliac branches (the aortoiliac bypass); or another operation to shunt blood through vein grafts or other conduits from the aorta to branches of the coronary arteries, in order to increase the flow beyond the local obstruction (the coronary bypass); or a third operation in which a vascular prosthesis is used to bypass an obstruction in the femoral artery where the graft may be synthetic material such as Dacron, or autologous tissue such as bovine carotid artery (the femoropopliteal bypass).

The coronary bypass is the most popular chest surgery done today. It takes tremendous skill, much training, and a large investment in the surgeon's education, along with some highly sophisticated and costly equipment supplied by the hospital involved. The whole procedure must go quickly and cleanly with great efficiency of motion and time. Every health professional involved works as part of the team.

Dr. Harper describes the Spokane hospital operation as among the most efficient. "First you receive an arteriogram [angiogram]; then a shave and cleaning of the chest. The anesthesiologist arrives and the operation begins," says Dr. Harper. "The surgeon's first cut is made before an hour and a half has passed."

Medical specialists shunt your blood to oxygenate it while your heart lies exposed. This is *the cardiopulmonary bypass*, a method of maintaining extracorporeal circulation by diversion of the blood flow away from the heart; blood is passed through a pump oxygenator (heart-lung machine) and then returned to the arterial side of the circulation.

Consider what might have happened tō you just a few hours before, suggests Dr. Harper as he sets the scene. Luckily the pain struck when your family was there and someone called for help. The ambulance with red light flashing and siren screaming rushed you to the big sterile building. At the hospital they didn't even ask what was wrong but wheeled you directly to the cardiopulmonary laboratory. There, some masked and white-coated doctor cut into your arm or leg under a local anesthetic and pushed a catheter through the vein into your heart. A technician took X-ray pictures as dye traveled through. The films were developed.

"Just sit there," you were told as they went into the hallway to speak with the little woman.

Your wife stands there wringing her hands and being brave.

"Your husband has had a heart attack," says the doctor. "He shows an abnormal angiogram. Come right in here and we'll show you the pictures. There! See how this artery is blocked and that artery is blocked? Your husband must have surgery immediately! Here is the operating permit to sign; he's not capable of signing."

In shock, the little woman asks, "Well, what if . . . what if he doesn't have the surgery?"

"He'll die! Your husband won't have enough oxygen to his heart tissue to live until morning."

She signs and you undergo a $25,000 operation within the next ninety minutes.

Hazards and Risks of Coronary Angiography

According to Dr. Harper, open heart surgery in Spokane, Washington is not predicated on the various enzyme studies usually employed and which are counted on to show abnormalities twelve to twenty-four hours after a heart attack occurs. And all cardiac attacks don't record on the EKG (electrocardiogram), so that even if your EKG is normal you may be operated upon. The operation's sole criterion to be performed in Spokane is angiogram — even though chest pain can come from pleurisy, pneumonia, muscle spasm, or even anxiety. There are many causes other than coronary occlusion. Have a chest complaint and get an angiogram!

Coronary angiography, also known as *arteriography*, involves passing a catheter into the heart under fluoroscopic control, and injecting radiopaque contrast material through the catheter into the coronary arteries. Films of the dye flowing through the coronary arteries can demonstrate narrowing or complete obstruction.

The technique has been extremely beneficial for diagnosis in the hands of a highly skilled physician-technologist. It has its hazards when the technician is not so skilled. Angiography is used to determine whether coronary artery surgery is indicated, especially in those people who suffer with severe disabling angina pectoris unresponsive to medical therapy. It may be useful also as a diagnostic determinant for preoperative evaluation for valvular surgery, and only *occasionally* for patients with recent myocardial infarction. A primary rule in the use of angiography is that the benefit of its use must outweigh its risks.[1]

Some clinicians use arteriography to diagnose or exclude coronary artery disease in patients unlikely to be considered for surgery, while others consider the procedure too hazardous for such "routine" diagnostic use.[2] Most physicians, however, will employ the procedure for patients only when surgery is contemplated, since it is relatively hazardous.

The death rate for angiography varies from 0.1 percent to 1.0 percent, depending on who is the doctor, how old and healthy is the patient, and whether the mortality statistic takes into account the patient's death at the time of procedure or six months later from an embolism sustained when the angiogram was performed. At any rate, the procedure may result in death, myocardial infarction, stroke, cerebral emboli, arrhythmias, thrombosis, arterial tear, and dissection at the site of arterial puncture.[3]

"The procedure is hazardous," says *The Medical Letter*, and warns against its overuse as a diagnostic test.[2] *The Medical Letter* offers information about drugs and therapeutics. It provides no-holds-barred commentary about the newest in medicine. Written by a bevy of renowned medical experts in many fields, it is sent to subscribing physicians.

Using arteriography, or angiography, as the sole criterion for determining surgical correction of coronary artery lesions seems unsound. Besides, the X-ray films are sometimes difficult to read, particularly when the patient is obese, and even experienced cardiologists and radiologists may differ in their interpretations.[4] Additionally, perfect human specimens at age forty who run five miles every morning and can conquer treadmill tests of 185 heart beats a minute will still frequently show documented abnormal angiograms (as much as fifty percent of healthy volunteers in a study) with fifty percent narrowing of the arterial lumen at age forty. Even so, the last thing the patient may need is dangerous heart surgery.

The New Medical-Surgical Fad

Just as there are medical differences of opinion about the benefits and risks of coronary arteriography, the same situation exists for that other potentially more dangerous vascular procedure, surgical bypass. *Coronary artery surgery*, also known as *bypass surgery*, is supposed to improve coronary circulation. It is a controversial, expensive, and extensive operation which has still not proven its value. Possibly coronary artery surgery has some value for relieving severe heart pain, but for only a limited number of patients with a narrow range of coronary conditions. Or possibly it might be used for relief of severe heart pain which fails to respond to medical therapy, including chelation therapy. Nevertheless, 80,000 people a year in more than 500 hospitals are undergoing open heart surgery. Introduced in the late 1960s, it has become the new medical-surgical fad for supposed repair of coronary arteries. The reason? Most of those undergoing surgery are told there are no alternatives. Do it or die!

James O. Stallings, M.D., a plastic surgeon of Des Moines, Iowa, told me, "The scar of open-heart surgery has become a kind of status symbol." In the minds of upward climbers, he said, a scar on the chest seems to have become a sign of social standing and the ultimate consequence of a life of hard work. It supposedly shows sacrifice to one's job and disregard of one's person for the building of a business.

Patients Take High Risks

Increasing numbers of patients without anginal pain or any other coronary symptoms are having clogged arteries bypassed in the hope of delaying a fatal heart attack. Yet there is virtually no evidence at all to support this hope. Patients accept high risks. They take as high as a twelve percent chance of inducing a heart attack due to the surgery — during or immediately after the operation. The 20-30 percent reocclusion rate of their graft in the next two years also must be considered.

The explosive growth in the last eight years of open-heart surgical facilities has raised serious questions about the adequacy of health care planning and controls in the way doctors are creating a demand for this possibly unnecessary surgery. The underlying reason for the surgery's overuse is because it is profitable. Are the doctors offering reasonable disclosures of the risks and the alternatives? In her book, *The Unkindest Cut*, Marcia Millman declares that they are not.[5]

Chelation therapy aside, critics of the bypass procedure say that many individuals may have their angina relieved by proper medication, weight loss, and a cessation of smoking. The National Heart, Lung and Blood Institute reported on March 9, 1977 that many patients with unstable angina responded well to drug treatment and had fewer heart attacks after therapy than those who underwent bypass surgery. And angina accounts for more than 75 percent of the bypass operations performed.

Henry D. McIntosh, M.D. of the Methodist Hospital in Houston, Texas said at a symposium of the American Heart Association in Miami Beach that bypass surgery should be reserved for patients with *crippling* angina who did not respond to more conservative treatment. "I do not believe that surgery is indicated for the asymptomatic patient," Dr. McIntosh said.[6] His comments are totally supported by the National Institutes of Health in its study.

Open-Heart Surgery Is Enormously Profitable

"Every time a surgeon does a heart bypass," suggests a health-care-delivery analyst, "he takes home a luxury sports car." The busy cardiac surgeon can easily earn over half-a-million dollars a year doing bypass procedures. By 1986, if enthusiasts of the operation have their way, hospitals and doctors will collect $100 billion a year doing just this one type of surgery.[5] American taxpayers will be responsible for making most of those payments. We already have paid out $3 billion in charges for open heart surgery performed just in 1976. Medicare picks up the tab on those over age sixty-five. The operations cost about $10,000 apiece for surgeons fees and $10,000 to $20,000 each for hospital expense.

"Yes, it's expensive," admitted heart surgeon W. Gerald Austen, M.D. of Massachusetts General Hospital in Boston. Then he sounded a warning, "We have to be careful of overly expanding its use."

Opponents say many of the operations are needless, that doctors are cashing in on a lucrative practice, which in turn encourages too many hospitals to invest in facilities that drive up health costs. Greater numbers of smaller hospitals throughout the country which seek more prestige in their communities are developing the extensive and expensive laboratory and surgical facilities and the medical teams needed to do coronary bypass surgery. Then, to justify the expenditures, keep beds filled, and maintain an appropriate level of staff skill, the hospitals must do several hundred such operations a year. The result is that they go looking for more patients. Knowing this, you can better understand why you should not get chest pains in a place like Spokane, Washington.

Tremendous financial outlays in surgical facilities are likely to create prejudice in favor of using them. This could inadvertently represent a powerful vested interest group among physicians who might feel threatened by an office procedure treatment that avoids the need for up to ninety percent of these surgeries. Such situations involving conflicts of interest do exist, as I shall describe in Chapter Fourteen.

Teamwork and Attention Are Required

The key to technical excellence for the bypass procedure, as mentioned previously, is expert medical teamwork and careful anesthesia. The operation takes an average of three hours. Sections of the saphenous vein in the leg are removed and sewn to the aorta at one end and coronary arteries at the other end. These attachments bypass parts of coronary arteries that are severely or totally obstructed, which ordinarily would supply the heart muscle with oxygen that it needs to pump effectively. During the operation, the patient's circulation is temporarily taken over by a heart-lung machine.

Before surgery, the status of the patient's coronary blood vessels must be evaluated by angiogram. As I already have said, this involves injecting a dye and inserting a catheter in the vessels to determine which arteries are blocked and to what extent. About two patients in every 1,000 die as a result of the evaluation procedure itself. Others are disabled by resulting complications with about an over-all one-percent complication incidence. Those are very real hazards of angiography, which usually must be done before bypass surgery.

The individual's survival after surgical bypass also depends largely on astute postoperative nursing in a coronary care unit, where potentially fatal complications can be detected and treated.

This type of teamwork and attention before, during, and after surgery calls for big money paid by the patient or his health insurance carrier. It would not be such a terribly high price to pay if coronary artery bypass really cured heart disease or prolonged life at least a little. It does neither. What does the surgery accomplish? It temporarily relieves chest pain symptoms — maybe — if the operation doesn't first kill the patient.

Complications that Result from Coronary Bypass Surgery

The purpose of coronary artery surgery is to improve the coronary circulation by graft insertion, but five to twenty-five percent of the grafts become occluded within a year.[7, 8] And up to thirty percent reocclude in two years. Whether the grafts become occluded or not, after months or years pain may recur with progression of atherosclerosis, reports Paul L. Tecklenberg, M.D. of Stanford University School of Medicine.[9] Some patients are advised to undergo a second coronary artery operation when angina pain returns.[10] The *patient* usually meekly assumes the blame for the failure of the surgery. He knows that he did not alter his style of living after the surgery, which he thought had made him "safe." Therefore, the surgeon is seldom blamed for those treatment failures, says author Marcia Millman.[5] Her book, *The Unkindest Cut*, is an indictment of medical cupidity in exploitation of patients. The coronary artery bypass procedure is one of the methods of that exploitation, she says.

Coronary artery bypass operations sometimes done as an emergency in patients with myocardial infarction can produce operative mortality rates as high as thirty percent.[11] The death rate from the operation varies, however, with the number of procedures performed at a given facility. For example,

Thomas Chalmers, M.D. of the Mount Sinai Medical Center in New York City pointed out in 1972 that surgical reports indicate a mortality rate of twelve percent for hospitals that perform 100 or fewer operations annually; reports of 100 to 200 cases performed annually at a facility indicate a nine percent death rate; when 200 or more cases are operated in the same surgical facility by its "team," the average mortality rate for the year drops to 4.5 percent.

Additionally, operative mortality for patients with congestive heart failure may be as high as 23 percent. [12] When the very severe complication known as *cardiogenic shock* strikes, the coronary artery surgical bypass patient death rate approaches 70 percent. [13]

All of this mortality connected with coronary artery bypass surgery certainly makes the opponents of chelation therapy sound downright silly. They dwell on the less than ten deaths over thirty-five years in which chelation therapy *may* be implicated, out of thousands of patients who have been helped, while no one stops to mention the thousands of deaths directly and unequivocally due to unproven bypass surgery.

A nonfatal complication of surgical bypass includes *perioperative infarction*, which is a reocclusion around the operative sites where the graft splices were made. This happens in as many as twenty percent of patients. [14, 15] Some pateints also experience arrhythmias, persistent postoperative bleeding, pulmonary complications, and infection. A major reason for complication with reinfarction to take place among coronary bypassed patients is that the same conditions exist in their bodies after the surgery, as prevailed before.

"The basic reasons for these people to have arteriosclerosis in the first place still persist," says Yiwen Y. Tang, M.D., chelation therapist of San Francisco. "Even one of the first heart transplant patients, a dentist named Philip Bleiberg, operated on by South African heart surgeon Dr. Christian N. Barnard in 1967, was reported to have died of coronary thrombosis after eighteen months. In other words, the patient received a new, young heart but became sick and died of used, old arteries. Not his doctor or anybody else bothered to help him change his lifestyle."

Coronary Bypass Fails to Prolong Life

What Dr. Tang has pointed out may explain the lack of prolonged life for heart transplant patients and coronary bypass patients.

According to the Organ Transplant Registry of the National Institutes of Health, only about twenty percent of human heart transplant patients survive longer than one year. And patients treated with coronary bypass surgery, compared to those treated with drugs, showed no evidence of increased survival or lowered risk of heart attack as a result of the surgery. [16,17]

One randomized trial in forty patients with acute coronary insufficiency involving various coronary vessels compared medical with surgical management; patients who had operations had higher functional capacity four months later, but differences in mortality were higher for them.[18]

More extensive controlled clinical trials comparing medical and surgical therapy are now underway. They are carefully designed by experts and are sponsored by the Veterans Administration and the National Heart, Lung and Blood Institute.[19,20,21] The studies are being undertaken to evaluate the benefits and risks of bypass surgery. All of the results won't be available for about five years, by which time more than 100,000 persons a year are likely to undergo the operation. These studies, although welcomed by medical researchers, are described by some as too slow in starting, especially in view of the enthusiasm that has surrounded bypass surgery since it was first described in the medical literature in 1970.

To date, significant differences in mortality between the medical management of occluded coronary arteries and surgical management by means of the bypass operation have *not* been reported, except for that March 9, 1977 announcement by the National Heart, Lung and Blood Institute. Michael B. Mock, M.D., the Institute's project officer for its study, said that in four years, doctors at eight medical centers across the country tested 288 patients. Of these, 147 received intensive drug therapy and 141 underwent bypass surgery. Mortality in the hospital after treatment was 4.1 percent for the medical group and 5 percent for the surgical patients. In follow-up studies averaging twenty-four months, medical group mortality was 5 percent against 5.2 percent among surgical patients. In the period of hospitalization, 10 percent of the medically treated group suffered heart attacks against 18 percent of the bypass patients.[22]

The Medical Letter said, "Although coronary artery surgery may relieve pain in patients with refractory disabling angina, it remains to be established whether coronary bypass operations improve long-term survival."[2]

Surgeons say they are successful in relieving pain in more than 75 percent of patients with disabling angina. The surgeons also admit that studies have yet to indicate that this operation prolongs life. The relief alone justifies operating, they say.

"There is a question whether the quantity of life will be improved, but there is no question that quality of life is improved," Dr. McIntosh said.[5]

Life's Quality After Surgical Bypass Is Questionable

Contrary to Dr. McIntosh's declaration, there is every kind of question about the quality of life after coronary artery surgical bypass. A previous surgery for heart disease called *the Internal Mammary Artery Ligation* was abandoned after it was conclusively demonstrated that the operation's relief of angina was all "placebo effect." Some physicians suspect that same placebo effect is partially responsible for the "benefits" of today's popular bypass surgery.

"Many patients do receive pain relief, but the relief is likely to come from the death of the symptomatic area from the heart attack induced at the time of the surgery with subsequent replacement of the area by a scar," Harold W. Harper, M.D. suggested to me.

"There is also an interruption of the nerve bundle that passes to the affected area of the heart. The pain receptor nerves are severed. As a result, no warning pain is present to signal when the heart is ischemic," he said.

Lucien Campeau, M.D., chief of cardiology at the Montreal Heart Institute, Montreal, Quebec, Canada, studied 235 patients angiographically one year after their coronary artery bypass operations. He split them into two groups: those operated on between October 1969 and September 1971, and between October 1971 and September 1973. During those intervals Dr. Campeau found the patient's graft opening had improved from 60 percent to 80 percent. But three years after surgery half of those same patients again studied by Dr. Campeau had no grafts remaining open. Even so, many of the closed-graft patients reported being improved or angina-free.[23]

"This unexpected pain relief may be the result of a 'pain-denial placebo effect,' " Dr. Campeau said. He confirmed what I implied earlier: The mere knowledge that they had undergone such a risky and expensive operation may be the cause of the patient's denying the sensation of pain, even if it actually is still present.

Then there are other explanations for no pain. Dr. Campeau said, "These patients may be getting better medical therapy. They're encouraged to stop smoking and lose weight. Many do not resume the same activity after surgery, and many are less anxious because of the operation."

Dr. Campeau cautions that there are implications for patients that are serious. Just as Dr. Harper mentioned, Dr. Campeau said, "Not having pain and yet having ischemia might jeopardize patients because they have lost the alarm of pain and might lead too active a life. If they have a positive stress test and still say that they are angina-free," he advises, "they should be watched more closely."

Thus the quality of life after coronary bypass surgery *seems* to improve when in reality this does not mean the patient has been *truly* benefited. The patient may only think he is restored to health and is lured to his death through over-exercise, suggested Ara G. Tilkian, M.D. of the Palo Alto, California, Veteran's Administration Hospital. Without the chest pain, Dr. Tilkian said, a person can sometimes over-exercise himself into new problems.

Exercise which is too severe can cause bypass surgical patients to develop arrhythmias, or irregular heart beats. "In our studies, one man got a lethal level of arrhythmias," said Dr. Tilkian. The absence of the chest pain removes a natural limiting factor.

Why Coronary Bypass Gets Heavy Referrals

I pointed out earlier that the surgical bypass for coronary arteries costs $25,000, more or less, including hospitalization, anesthesiologists' fees, surgeons' fees, and other expenses. It has a high mortality rate. It may reduce the incidence of chest pain but fails to prolong a person's life. The surgery does not cure atherosclerosis, which is a chronic progressive disease. It only grafts a substitute blood vessel which is a vein, not an artery, as a replacement for an occluded artery. Thus the substitute blood vessel is thinner and more prone to develop disease. Furthermore, this is treatment for only a single arterial segment. All the rest of the arterial system is affected by the same problems. Toxic materials remain present in the bloodstream and vessels, but they are left untreated.

Nonetheless, with all of these disadvantages, the many hazards and risks connected with coronary artery bypass, a lot of physicians recommend their patients have this operation. Why? Why are doctors willing to put their patients' lives in jeopardy for so little lasting benefit? I know of at least two major reasons.

Heavy referrals come from some physicians who have been led to believe that not much can be done for angina victims. They try arterial dilating agents first, such as nitroglycerine, papaverine, propanolol, and perhaps a hundred other drugs of this type that are medically marketed. Then the doctors may give up on the vasodilators and move to blood thinners such as coumadin and other medications. One of the marks in medicine of a therapy being ineffective is that there are so many different drugs to treat the same problem. If drugs were specific and effective, there would be a need for only one.

The arterial dilating agents in general cannot work. They cannot stretch, or make larger, a blood vessel that has a calcium-lined wall. The arterial wall is hardened, diseased, and scarred. The dilators will work only on those arterial segments that are undiseased. Their action, therefore, primarily may be psychological. They have a placebo effect for the patient and give the physician a little soothing for his own conscience by his trying to accomplish something — anything — for an otherwise hopeless disease. Most physicians finally realize, sadly, that they are unable to do very much for their arteriosclerotic patients. This realization is very hard on the average doctor's ego, as it reminds him of how truly impotent he really is.

Consequently, even those physicians who are conscientious and empathetic, have the compulsion to get the hopeless patients with really severe angina off their hands. Also many doctors don't know the true statistics of failure for bypass surgery. They treat severe heart cases with standard drugs that are extremely limited. Such frustrated physicians are forced finally to sweep these personally discomforting patients under the therapeutic rug — out of their practices and into the hands of vascular surgeons or chest surgeons or others who perform open-heart surgery.

The second major reason for heavy referrals to open-heart surgeons is the better financial return for referring cardiologists. They collect larger and more frequent fees to carry out pre-operative and post-operative procedures on surgical in-hospital patients than to manage strictly medical therapy. Also, health insurance carriers seem to pay on policies more readily to cardiologists when chest surgery is involved.

Surgical Bypass Is Controversial

If physicians were more selective about their referrals and sent only the sickest patients for surgical repair, the bypass procedure would not be so controversial. But the heart surgeons are careful to take only healthy candidates, such as forty-year-olds with a little chest pain and a slightly irregular electrocardiogram. They will not take on a desperate patient who might increase an individual surgeon's death score. That kind of seriously ill patient is denied surgery and seldom is informed of the chelation alternative. The only answer is a shrug of the shoulders by the surgeon and his admonition, "You are not a surgical bypass candidate." The really desperate patient is left to wait and wonder and. . . .[24, 31]

Even for someone previously accepted for heart surgery, he or she is often refused for later repeated bypass attempts no matter how seriously ill the person is now. The heart surgeons guard their patient mortality rates against expansion but not necessarily out of humanitarian motives. Recently, the president-elect of the American College of Chest Surgeons was asked to step aside and not take office because he had a 51 percent surgical mortality rate among his patients. He would have given the chest surgeons a bad name, they explained. He apparently did not turn down these more advanced high risk cases as regularly and studiously as had his fellow surgeons.

We see than that selection of patients is biased in favor of good surgical results. Not just anybody can have a coronary bypass. The heart surgeons prefer not to add onto their mortality scores. They accept only those people they believe will have a high survival rate. Worst of all, many patients are even encouraged to have chest surgery "prophylactically." This is wonderful for the surgeon, since these have the best survival rates and keep his mortality statistics looking good. It is a big moneymaker in medicine with elaborate facilities and highly trained personnel that have to be kept hard at work. The huge investment won't permit otherwise.

The Chelation Therapy Contrast

Arteriosclerotic vascular disease is not a segmental disease. Medical science has shown in repeated studies that the condition does not affect only individual arteries, such as the coronaries around the heart, the carotids leading to the brain, or the aorta and femorals leading to the legs. It affects the entire body everywhere, particularly wherever there is an arterial bifurcation (a division or offshoot of the artery).

Unlike surgery which cannot be done on the smaller and frequently inaccessible blood vessels, the arterioles and the capillaries, chelation therapy does reach the tiny occluded segments along with the larger occluded ones. The entire arterial system and all the cells of the body have toxic minerals removed by EDTA infusion. Basic causes are thus treated. The load on the heart is reduced by lowering the resistance to blood flow. Anytime flow resistance in the arterial system is reduced, the heart is required to work less hard to accomplish the same job. Other problem areas improve, including a lowering of insulin requirements for diabetics, a decrease in elevated blood pressure, a fall in excess serum cholesterol and triglycerides, reduced senility, more mobility for arthritic joints, and many other improvements.

Bypass surgery performed in the limbs, the heart, or anywhere in the body comes nowhere near providing the beneficial effects of EDTA chelation therapy. Chelation apparently does prolong life and does heighten the quality of life. Its cost is usually less than ten percent of the expense of bypass surgery.

Finally, despite the heart surgeon's common claim that he has never heard of the treatment or that it could not help, chelation therapy has often come to the aid of those whom the surgeons failed to help. Or it has provided new life to people who were so far advanced in their disease they decided against even trying surgery.

Chapter Eleven

The Medical Controversy over EDTA Chelation Therapy

The medical mystique has its own rules and regulations. Many have a compelling logic and are judiciously applied. But some of them ought to be questioned. The central question is whether the rules are used to promote the therapeutic aspects of the medical mystique, or whether they are employed to reinforce the mystique's authoritarian aspects. . . Hippocrates, in his oath, speaks not just of taking care of patients, but of the obligations of all new members to their teachers. And Fellows. Most lay people think of the Hippocratic Oath as a dedication to the patient. But the oath also clearly defines what a doctor's obligations are to other members of the profession.
— Marvin S. Belsky, M.D. and
Leonard Gross, *How to Choose
and Use Your Doctor*, 1975

The Anti-Chelation CMA Resolution 151-73

Reference Committee D-1 of the California Medical Association House of Delegates met February 23, 1975 to consider Resolution 151-75 on chelation therapy, as part of its studies on "Scientific and Educational Activities." Resolution 151-75, introduced by Wayne B. Bigelow, M.D. of Turlock, California, representing the Stanislaus County Medical Society, declared:

WHEREAS, Chelation has been demonstrated by the FDA to be dangerous and
WHEREAS, its effectiveness has not been established in arteriosclerotic disease, be it
RESOLVED: that the use of Chelation be limited to research centers until further data is available.

Communications consultant Phil Townsend Hanna, a legislative advocate for the Committee for Medical Freedom, 1127 Eleventh St., Suite 501, Sacramento, California, was an observer at the committee meeting. Mr. Hanna reported that Dr. Bigelow, who assists in doing coronary artery bypass surgery, stated he was "unfamiliar with the general aspects of chelation therapy except for its use to remove heavy metals." Dr. Bigelow had introduced his antichelation resolution on his own, without first clearing it with the Scientific Committee of the California Medical Association

(CMA). Then he agreed that his resolution should be rewritten to exclude this use in heavy metal poisoning. Dr. Bigelow said he knew of several clinics which were formed or were being formed to deal exclusively in chelation therapy for arteriosclerotic diseases. He complained to the reference committee that patients were being charged "high fees" for this unproved treatment, and that the Food and Drug Administration did not approve of its use for this purpose. (The FDA does not "approve" of many treatments commonly employed by medical doctors.)

Ralph C. Teall, M.D. of Sacramento, California rose to support Dr. Bigelow's resolution. Dr. Teall is a former vice president of the American Medical Association and full-time acting medical director for the California-Western States Life Insurance Company, which is controlled by the Occidental Life Insurance Company. The Occidental Life Insurance Company is the Medicare health insurance carrier for Southern California. Dr. Teall said that he had researched chelation and there was nothing whatsoever to support its use. Even as he spoke, however, Dr. Teall had on his reference committee desk two recently published Russian articles. [1,2] Both articles reported beneficial effects on cerebral, coronary and peripheral circulation on all the patients studied with use of EDTA, as well as with another chelating agent, Unithiol, which employes a sulfhydryl group as the chelator. [3]

Dr. Teall also said a doctor in Sacramento (meaning Garry F. Gordon, M.D.) operated a chelation therapy clinic. (The Sacramento Medical Preventics Clinic is a private health care facility engaged in the active application of preventive medicine concepts within a holistic framework. Dr. Gordon gave up his affiliation with the clinic when he assumed duties as president of the American Academy of Medical Preventics in September 1976.) This doctor, said Dr. Teall, was supporting a staff with an annual payroll of more than $600,000.

Then Dr. Teall described the heated legal battle between the chelation therapy clinic and the Sacramento Medical Care Foundation, which had rejected the clinic's insurance claims. The clinic had brought suit and an injunction against the Sacramento Medical Care Foundation. For the first time in California history, depositions were taken in open court before a judge, said Dr. Teall.

This insurance company medical director also warned his colleagues that other clinics were being formed for this chelation treatment. He said that the Sacramento doctor was being bankrolled by other doctors from all over the country. Dr. Teall emphasized that various patients were being sold a bill of goods and lulled into believing the efficacy of the treatment with "literature that was old." To his knowledge, he told the committee, nothing new had been printed on the subject since 1963 (while the pro-chelation articles *on his desk* had been published in 1972 and 1973.)

What Dr. Teall did *not* tell the members of the CMA's Reference Committee D-1 was possibly the real reason for his interest in having this anti-chelation resolution passed. The CMA could take the blame while his insurance company refused to pay potential health insurance claims for reimbursement by patients who were being treated in Dr. Gordon's clinic or in other chelation facilities. The resolution's passage would give Dr. Teall's employer a valid excuse to deny payments.

Franklin Ashley, M.D., a member of the Scientific Board of the California Medical Association, stood up to support the Bigelow resolution. He claimed the CMA needed to run the charlatans and thieves out of the medical profession, and that none of the information on chelation therapy for arteriosclerosis had even been presented to the CMA Scientific Board.

Leonard Asher, M.D. from the Los Angeles delegation added that CMA should do something to inform the AMA and the public about this type of treatment which was not approved by the FDA.

The CMA Reference Committee D-1 then took the matter under submission when no one rose in opposition to the House of Delegates Resolution 151-75. No one was present from the American Academy of Medical Preventics (AAMP) who could have presented the facts in defense of chelation therapy, because the Academy members were *not* informed of the pending resolution. And there was no known opposition when the CMA House of Delegates voted to approve the following amended resolution:

> RESOLVED: That the CMA opposes the use of chelation therapy in the treatment of arteriosclerotic disease except in recognized research centers; and, be it further
> RESOLVED: That the CMA inform physicians and the public of the documented dangers and lack of proven benefit of chelation therapy as a treatment for arteriosclerotic diseases.

Effects of the Resolution's Adoption

The resolution warns against "documented dangers." This stems from the EDTA overdosage in two patients in 1954, reported in 1955, that I told you about in Chapter Seven. Dr. Clarke's explanation and Dr. Halstead's interpretation of those overdosages with EDTA were presented then. More than two million treatments on many thousands of patients have been given since 1954 with no reports of deleterious results.

The resolution also charges "lack of proven benefit." But what is the proof required? Over and over, published clinical journal articles report chelated patients whose electrocardiograms (EKGs) get better; their plethysmographs improve. They can walk where they could not before receiving chelation therapy. Patients don't die! What more proof has been needed in medicine until now?

Resolution 151-75 was introduced into the House of Delegates of the CMA with no thought to its fairness. It went through as a matter of routine and became the rule of the California state medical society.

Effects of the resolution's adoption filtered down to the general CMA membership quickly. A sixty-eight-year-old physician in Northern California, who is a benevolent person supporting his twelve adopted children, received a telephone call declaring that he was being kicked out of his local medical society because he was a chelating doctor. He was losing all the professional and economic advantages of membership. Almost immediately his professional life began to decline. A distinct loss of respect from his fellow physicians was felt by him almost at once. Worse still, his medical malpractice insurance, disability insurance, health insurance, hospital insurance, and life insurance were being cancelled. He had purchased these various insurance coverages through the CMA's group plans, which were part of the benefits of medical society membership.

Without a hearing, with no due process, he was told, "You are out!" Consequently, under pressure the physician signed a paper which read in part: "I hereby promise not to use chelation therapy. . . "

Harvard University medical graduate Yiwen Y. Tang, M.D., F.A.B.F.P. of San Francisco, received a similar declaration by mail from the San Francisco Medical Society. He was threatened with expulsion unless he stopped using chelation therapy. Dr. Tang's response was not one of anxiety or fear but of anger. He telephoned Garry F. Gordon, M.D. and said, "We can't let this go on. We have to stand up and be counted!"

Dr. Gordon agreed. "Let's call their bluff," he said and gathered together the defense forces of the 300-member American Academy of Medical Preventics.

The American Academy of Medical Preventics (with executive offices at 305 S. Doheny Drive, Beverly Hills, California 90211; (213) 878-1234; Lynne Stone, executive director), is a professional organization formed for the research and development of the clinical applications of any vascular therapy. It educates physicians and the public about cardiovascular disease and the application of chelation to that disease. The Academy also works toward the widespread recognition of vitamin/mineral supplementation, diet modification, anti-stress factors, exercise, and other changes in lifestyles that might alter the course of this disease.

AAMP is attempting to do basic research and has contacted the FDA to explore the possibility of proceeding with clinical testing of EDTA under a physician-sponsored IND (Investigational New Drug Application). Academy members hope to see EDTA moved from "possibly effective" to "proven effective" for the purposes of FDA regulations. Unfortunately, this seemingly simple task appears virtually impossible for a small group of private physicians. Estimates at potential cost vary from $500,000 to $5 million. Apparently, pressure must be applied before government funds are put to this use. This requires informed people who will write their representatives in Washington to request such research funding.

AAMP member physicians use alternative cardiovascular therapies that involve early detection, identifying the risk factors of the patient, and then intensive education in modifying the patient's lifestyle to alter those risk factors. Chelation therapy may be employed to further modify the course of the patient's disease process before it reaches crisis proportions. As a result, there may be substantial early treatment for large numbers of patients and little need for vascular or other bypass surgery later.

These AAMP physicians practice *holistic preventive medicine*. The holistic approach is a full program that dedicates itself to reversal of our major killer disease, hardening of the arteries, and other diseases. A referral list of physician members in various parts of the country is maintained by the organization. To learn of a physician near you who uses rehabilitative exercise, nutritional therapy, and chelation therapy against arteriosclerosis, write to the American Academy of Medical Preventics at the Beverly Hills address.

The AAMP versus the CMA

The San Francisco Medical Society conducted a peer review of their "errant" member. Dr. Tang went to the committee meeting with two slide projectors full of "before and after" slides of his patients' chelation treatment results (see Dr. Tang's photographs 1, 2, 3, 4 of Roland Hohnbaum in Chapter One). He also supplied quantities of the basic medical journal documents which his San Francisco colleagues apparently had never seen. He said, "Gentlemen, you are interested in chelation; you wish to know about it; now you are going to learn."

Dr. Tang was an hour and a half into his peer review presentation when the committee chairman noted that more than half of his committee members had left. They had come to censor their colleague and not to learn from him. The chairman was embarrassed and called a halt to the documentation. Dr. Tang then handed the peer review chairman a letter prepared in advance. The letter read:

> Yiwen Y. Tang, M.D., Inc.
> 345 Portal Avenue
> San Francisco, California 94118
> Telephone (415) 566-1000

San Francisco Medical Society
Professional Relations Committee
250 Masonic Ave.
San Francisco, California 84118

Sirs:

As a member of this medical society and as a physician whose practice includes the use of EDTA Chelation Therapy, I am requesting formally that my Society initiate action to rectify a serious error on the part of our parent organization, the California Medical Association. Specifically, I am referring to the CMA's resolution, passed in February of this year, which effectively proscribes the clinical use of EDTA Chelation Therapy. The language of that resolution claims that the Federal FDA has found chelation to be dangerous and unsubstantiated by scientific and clinical research. My personal documentation and the documentation of the American Academy of Medical Preventics (a professional society which specializes in Chelation Therapy and in which I am a member) overwhelmingly supports the opposite conclusions. In fact, correspondence with the FDA in no way supports the statement that chelation is dangerous.

I formally request you to determine on what basis this erroneous information was allowed to be introduced into a resolution and subsequently passed without prior notification to physicians who are engaged in the practice of chelation, of which there are approximately 120 in the State of California. The existence of the resolution threatens the availability of this modality to my patients and my particular practice of medicine. Since medical doctors in this state are being harassed by their local medical societies to discontinue this treatment for their patients or lose their society membership with the attendant loss of malpractice insurance, this resolution denies an effective alternative therapy in cardiovascular disease to the citizens of California. The "ban" on EDTA Chelation Therapy appears to have been initiated out of concern for potential costs to insurance carriers rather than concern for the health of people.

I request that some document signed by FDA showing EDTA to be dangerous be made available to myself, my Academy, and my patients. If such document cannot be produced, the faulty language must be brought to the attention of the CMA so that the unfortunate error can be corrected. Further, I request that proof regarding the alleged ineffectiveness of chelation be substantiated and made public to me, my Academy, and my patients. If such evidence cannot be provided, the CMA resolution must be rescinded as being without basis in fact.

The documentation which I presented to you tonight is overwhelmingly positive regarding EDTA's effectiveness in the removal of calcium in arteriosclerotic conditions in cadavers, experimental animals, and in living patients. I am appealing to your sense of objectivity and my rights to require proof of accusation. My actions here are in the best interest of The Society and medicine-at-large. . . .

Should you require additional information, please contact me directly.

Sincerely,
(signed)
Yiwen Y. Tang, M.D.

A letter arrived in Dr. Tang's office from Robert Mandle, M.D., Chairman of the Professional Relations Committee of the San Francisco Medical Society, four weeks after that meeting. It stated unceremoniously that Dr. Tang's letter had been taken under advisement. The San Francisco Medical Society would inform him of whatever action it took, the letter promised. Until this day, however, that letter from Dr. Mandle was the last Dr. Tang has heard from the San Francisco Medical Society.

Harassment continued for other chelating physicians in the State of

California. Some doctors considered giving up being crusaders for patients' rights. It was easier to abandon the fight and flow with the mainstream of "cookbook" medicine, a few decided. Therefore, on October 20, 1975 Dr. Tang and the AAMP filed a petition for a hearing before the Scientific Board of the California Medical Association. The hearing petition read:

To:
C. John Tupper, M.D.
Chairman, Scientific Board
California Medical Association
731 Market Street
San Francisco, California 94103

From:
Yiwen Y. Tang, M.D.
345 Portal Avenue
San Francisco, California 94118

and

American Academy of Medical
    Preventics
305 S. Doheny Drive
Beverly Hills, California 90211

On behalf of myself, my immediate colleagues and the American Academy of Medical Preventics, I HEREBY PETITION FOR A FORMAL HEARING BEFORE THE SCIENTIFIC BOARD BY VIRTUE OF THAT BOARD'S FUNCTION ACCORDING TO CHAPTER 4, SECTION 1, OF THE BY-LAWS OF THE CALIFORNIA MEDICAL ASSOCIATION.

Subject of the hearing is EDTA Chelation Therapy and the scientific basis thereof. Purpose of this hearing is to validate the right of the patient to receive this therapy, and the right of the physician who performs that modality to maintain his or her status as member in good standing of his local medical society and its related organizations. Specifically, we challenge the substance of CMA Resolution 151-75, which effectively proscribes Chelation Therapy to clinical practitioners who choose to use that treatment in arteriosclerotic diseases.

Passage of this resolution represents, in our opinion, a travesty of objective deliberation and due-process. . .

. . . .The proscription of EDTA Chelation Therapy was approved by the CMA under dubious conditions. There was no notification to practitioners in the field nor to our professional organization, all of whom were well known to all parties involved backing Resolution 151-75 before the CMA Reference Committee in Los Angeles. Thus, we seek a redress of due-process at the level of the Scientific Board, where the initial inquiries should have occurred in the first place, not in the political arena.

Resolution 151-75 was enacted by the CMA. It claimed that EDTA Chelation Therapy is dangerous, and that its efficacy has not been demonstrated. We are prepared to provide overwhelming evidence to the contrary on both points. For that purpose, then, we petition the following specific actions from the Scientific Board:

1. THAT WRITTEN ACKNOWLEDGEMENT OF THIS PETITION BE SENT BY REGISTERED MAIL WITHIN 15-DAYS FROM DATE OF DELIVERY TO THE OFFICES OF THE AMERICAN ACADEMY OF MEDICAL PREVENTICS (address above),

2.   THAT YOUR SCIENTIFIC BOARD MAKE A DETAILED AND COM-
PLETE ANALYSIS OF THE SCIENTIFIC LITERATURE REGARDING CHE-
LATION THERAPY UPON WHICH RESOLUTION 151-75 WAS ENACTED,
AND IF THAT DATA IS INSUFFICIENT TO SUBSTANTIATE THE RESOLU-
TION ACCORDING TO ACCEPTABLE SCIENTIFIC CRITERIA, THAT YOU
INITIATE APPROPRIATE REMEDIAL PROCEDURES;

3.   THAT IF, IN YOUR OPINION, YOUR REVIEW OF THE DATA SUS-
TAINS THE RESOLUTION, YOU ISSUE A FORMAL REQUEST TO THE
CMA FOR A MORATORIUM ON THE ENFORCEMENT OF RESOLUTION
151-75 UNTIL OUR FULL RECOURSE HAS BEEN EXHAUSTED (such a
moratorium is not necessary if our requested hearing will be held within
60-days of this petition; otherwise we believe that the lives and health of our
patients are at risk);

4.   THAT, AS PART OF THIS RECOURSE, A FULL FORMAL HEARING BE
SCHEDULED WITH THE FULL SCIENTIFIC BOARD TO EVALUATE OFFI-
CIALLY THE TWO ISSUES WE ARE CONTESTING. THIS INCLUDES THE
TOXICITY OF EDTA AND ITS EFFICACY IN ARTERIOSCLEROSIS WHICH,
WE BELIEVE, IS SUFFICIENTLY ESTABLISHED AS AN ACCEPTABLE
MEDICAL TREATMENT IN RELATION TO EXISTING ALTERNATIVES
TODAY;

5.   THAT WE RECEIVE, 30 DAYS PRIOR TO ANY SCHEDULED HEARING,
A STATEMENT WHICH OUTLINES THE CRITERIA BY WHICH YOUR
BOARD, OR THE CMA, DETERMINES ANY THERAPY TO BE ACCEPT-
ABLE MEDICAL TREATMENT: THAT IF SUCH CRITERIA ARE NOT A
MATTER OF PUBLISHED POLICY, OR IF SUCH CRITERIA DO NOT EXIST,
WE REQUEST THAT WHATEVER STANDARDS ARE TO BE EMPLOYED IN
THIS INSTANCE BE DETAILED FOR US IN A WRITTEN STATEMENT
WHICH IS ENDORSED BY YOURSELF OR OTHER AUTHORITATIVE OF-
FICIAL SOURCE;

6.   THAT WE BE ALLOWED AT LEAST TEN EXPERT WITNESSES AND A
MINIMUM OF THREE HOURS TO MAKE OUR PRESENTATION: AND
THAT A TRANSCRIPTION OF THE ENTIRE PROCEEDINGS BE PERMIT-
TED SO THAT THE INFORMATION MAY BE MADE AVAILABLE TO IN-
TERESTED PARTIES.

The above concludes our formal petition. In the following section, we should like
to explore several relevant areas in order to amplify your general understanding of
the issues as we see them.

— — — — —

In reference to the specific allegation that EDTA is dangerous:

The toxicity of EDTA has been studied in depth and the literature is extensive on
this subject. The substance is essentially an innocuous chemical when administered in the currently accepted dosage schedules (3 grams over a 2-plus-hour
period is the standard protocol today). EDTA is a standard analytical chemical
extensively employed in laboratories and industry (it has been used to clean lime
deposits from the inside of boilers for years, and it is a common food preservative
— you eat it frequently). Its LD-50, in relation to therapeutic dose, is considerably
safer the aspirin. We are enclosing several relevant citations to this issue.

1. Meltzer, L. E., et al.
   "The Long Term Side Effects and Toxicity of Disodium Ethylenedi-amine Tetracetic Acid (EDTA)." *American Journal of Medical Sciences*, July, 1961.

2. Oser, B.
   "Safety Evaluation Studies of Calcium EDTA." *Toxicology and Applied Pharmacology* 5:142-162, 1963.

3. Doolan, P. D., et al.
   "An Evaluation of the Nephrotoxicity of Ethylene diamine tetraace-tate and Diethylene triamine pentaacetate in the Rat." *Toxicology and Applied Pharmacology* 10:481-500, 1967.

4. Foreman, H.
   "Toxic Side Effects of Ethylene diamine Tetraacetic Acid." *Journal of Chronic Disease* 16:319-323, 1963.

In reference to Dr. Teall's statement that nothing has been published since 1963 regarding EDTA's efficacy:

We would make reference to the Biological Abstracts, Medline Computer Retrieval, and particularly the citations published by the National Library of Medicine on EDTA from 1967 to 1970 which reports 517 citations alone. . . See also the Federal Register which lists EDTA as possibly effective in vascular occlusive disease.

A collateral issue in the controversy is the subject of the package insert. We all realize that in medicine, there are always proponents of particular therapeutic approaches, from psychiatry to acupuncture, who believe they demonstrate efficacy, and opponents who dispute the position. The lack of a specific indication on the package insert for vascular occlusive disease does not make its use unacceptable in medicine. In the case of EDTA, the package insert was removed voluntarily by Abbott several years ago when they were unable to justify the expense of proving their claim about efficacy in arteriosclerotic disease and in light of a rapidly expiring patent on the chemical. Package inserts have recently been the subject of concern of the AMA Board of Trustees, who have requested the FDA to put a disclaimer at the bottom of these inserts so that physicians would not feel so governed and limited by the listed indications. The use of Diphenylhydantoin for many therapeutic applications not mentioned on the package insert, as well as Propanolol Hydrochloride, must serve to remind us that the FDA has no jurisdiction over the practice of medicine, and its authority is concerned primarily with marketing claims — at least as far as the package insert is concerned. The FDA states that the use of a locally obtained drug in a physician's office is the "practice of medicine" over which they have no jurisdiction. See: R. Crout, M.D. *The Lowly Package Insert*, Dir. Bureau of Drugs — FDA.

The legal ramifications of the proscription against Chelation Therapy for arteriosclerosis by the CMA, although perhaps a more subtle issue, are potentially the most explosive. Every physician has the duty to disclose all available choices of therapy to the patient, and if he fails to do so, he may be held liable (ref. *Cobbs vs Grant* 8 Cal 3d 240, 104 C.R. 505). This might well be held applicable to a group or organization of physicians. We believe EDTA Chelation Therapy is a viable alternative in vascular disease for many patients and that it is significantly less dangerous than the alternatives made available at present.

There are other issues which are germane to this controversy, namely:

1. the current trend to politicize science and medicine, making certain therapies acceptable, such as acupuncture when sufficient public pressure is brought to bear, while other therapies are made illegal and their practitioners subject to arrest.

2. the subversion of organized medicine away from the role of protecting the rights of the patient to receive unfettered care of a physician who is practicing under his essentially unlimited license in California toward becoming the enforcer of "cost control medicine," etc. . . .

But these issues are not intended to be adjudicated by the Scientific Committee. Our fondest hope is that the name of science can be vindicated by objective evaluation instead of the sham of Resolution 151-75 being allowed to set the standard. We hope that we will not have to join the present exodus away from the organized medical institutions in the name of justice and fair treatment. This is a major responsibility on you as a representative of official judgment, but we are entering a period in which these issues are coming to a head across the nation and precedence must be established. The established institutions cannot continue to rule by fiat but must, instead, substantiate their positions in fact, upon reason, and in open forum. We trust that you are worthy of the task and, as a colleague in a tradition which transcends prejudice and ephemeral vested interest, we extend to you our firm regards.

Sincerely,

(signed)
Yiwen Y. Tang, M.D.

(signed)
Garry F. Gordon, M.D.
as Board Member and on behalf
of the American Academy of
Medical Preventics

Months passed during which the following actions took place:

November 17, 1975: The CMA replied to Dr. Tang with no mention of any acceptance of the conditions as requested in the petition.

November 26, 1975: CMA attorneys responded to Dr. Gordon's letter, which was mailed to them October 31, 1975. He requested resolution 151-75 be placed in moratorium until adequate hearing of the facts had been held. The attorneys answered, "CMA policy position is not a direct mandate which all physicians must follow." (Of course, if doctors don't follow it they apparently stand to lose their CMA membership and all related insurance benefits.)

December 1, 1975: The Federal Appeals Court in Atlanta, Georgia ruled that chelation therapy is a reasonable and necessary treatment and that Medicare Part A may pay Mr. D. D. Dominey for this treatment (as reported in Chapter Nine).

January 26, 1976: AAMP-Dr. Tang replied to the vague CMA November 17, 1975 letter and demanded again a *full and fair hearing in an open forum with recording of the entire proceedings.*

February 26, 1976: The CMA sent notice that it was granting a tape recorded hearing to Dr. Tang and the AAMP to be held at the Los Angeles Airport Marriott Hotel March 26, 1976 at 2:00 p.m.

With notice of a hearing to be held, the AAMP gathered together its witnesses and evidence of treatment efficacy. The Academy's relevant request was ignored, however, and at no time were any criteria by which EDTA could be found acceptable ever established by the CMA. The officers of AAMP submitted repeated written requests right up to the meeting-time for those guidelines. Also, no right to question the opponents of chelation therapy and force them to document their negative statements was granted. These denials or lack of actions constituted a serious disallowance of due-process on the part of the CMA. It foretold of the probable negative conclusion of the proceedings.

The CMA's Ad Hoc Committee Meeting

The hearing began as scheduled by an ad hoc committee of the *Advisory Panel on Internal Medicine of the Scientific Board of the California Medical Association*. It related to the resolution passed by the CMA's House of Delegates. "The Scientific Board and the House of Delegates are two clearly distinct and different organizations," said C. John Tupper, M.D., Chairman of the CMA Scientific Board. "The Scientific Board is responsible for the scientific and educational activities of the California Medical Association, and so quite separate."

In its attempt to prove the issues, the American Academy of Medical Preventics provided the CMA ad hoc committee with an enormous amount of medical documentation, plus color slides showing the beneficial effects of EDTA chelation. In verification, Dr. Tupper said, "I want you to know that we have received through Dr. Garry Gordon five boxes of reprints and other printed material that for your information weighs 102 pounds. We have them behind us here."

Although the AAMP members would have welcomed more time, in the three hours allowed it did furnish evidence for the following:

• EDTA is non-toxic when administered under proper medical supervision.

• EDTA is effective in the majority of cases of arteriosclerosis and its complications.

• Since arteriosclerosis is invariably fatal, compared with other presently used and acceptable modalities, the EDTA chelation therapy for arteriosclerosis has a very promising and highly acceptable benefit/risk ratio. In fact, the risk is exceedingly low and as such, constitutes an acceptable medical treatment for the palliation of arteriosclerosis and its complications.

Subsequent to its presentation, the AAMP urged the CMA Scientific Board's Advisory Panel to make a speedy decision to rescind Resolution 151-75 by the CMA House of Delegates, for the reasons indicated in its petition.

Following the AAMP three-hour presentation, another hour went by while the CMA ad hoc committee members randomly questioned the AAMP members. During their questioning, the CMA ad hoc committee presented no opponents of chelation therapy. Although the AAMP had petitioned for and expected to "meet with the appropriate panels in an open forum, face-to-face, for a free and open exchange of information" and to counter the arguments of medical opponents, none appeared. The notorized transcript of that hearing which I hold indicates that there was no exchange of information — only questions asked by the CMA and answers given by the AAMP.

It was anticipated by AAMP members that the open hearing would "provide both sides with better access to each other's information regarding the use of EDTA chelation therapy as a palliative in arteriosclerosis and enable our Academy [AAMP] to learn first hand of any information that you have that may indicate a possible danger or harmful effect of this therapy of which we are unaware, as well as the facts upon which any opposition is based. Possibly we may learn of an alternative therapy that offers equal opportunity for symptomatic relief in arteriosclerosis and which is less controversial." The CMA Scientific Board was unresponsive to this portion of the petition.

Dr. Gordon told me of an exchange between two CMA committee members overheard in the men's washroom by an AAMP member. It went like this.

"How long do we have to listen to this s**t?"

"Just long enough to let these idiots dump out their stuff. We'll soon get rid of them and finish them off."

Following the four-hour meeting, the CMA decision was seemingly arrived at within fifteen minutes. One of the AAMP medical witnesses, Lester I. Tavel, D.O. of Houston, Texas, had to catch a plane immediately at the conclusion of the meeting. He left for the airport, which was across the street, to check in for his flight. Fifteen minutes later he saw three of the CMA ad hoc committee members arrive at the airport bar. Each committee member had left behind at the place where he had been sitting his huge pile of exhibit and reference material supplied by the AAMP. And the CMA ad hoc committee of the Scientific Board never met again. Was this a "full and fair" hearing?

The CMA Ad Hoc Committee's Recommendation

The Advisory Panel on Internal Medicine and the Executive Committee of the Scientific Board April 14, 1976 endorsed the following recommendation to serve as official CMA policy regarding chelation therapy in the treatment of arteriosclerosis in lieu of House of Delegates Resolution 151-75:

> THE EFFICACY OF CHELATION THERAPY IN THE TREATMENT OF ARTERIOSCLEROSIS IS UNPROVEN AND IT IS NOT NOW AN ACCEPTED THERAPY. WHEN USED FOR SUCH TREATMENT, DISODIUM EDETATE (ENDRATE, EDTA) IS AN EXPERIMENTAL DRUG. THUS, THE CALIFORNIA MEDICAL ASSOCIATION RECOMMENDS THAT SUCH USE, IN EACH PATIENT, BE REPORTED TO THE FDA AND FURTHER, THAT IT REQUIRE THE PATIENT'S INFORMED CONSENT.

During the summer of 1976 newspapers around the country printed nearly similar stories that were critical of chelation therapy. They appeared in towns and cities where chelation physicians practiced and were adapted to include local or regional medical personnel in authority. The following article, from the *Salt Lake City Tribune* of August 8, 1976, is typical:

> The Salt Lake City-County Health Department has questioned the use of chelation therapy for arteriosclerosis and multiple sclerosis.
> Dr. Harry L. Gibbons, city-county health director said there is inadequate evidence that chelation therapy, which uses trace metal elements in a nutrient solution may be beneficial to arteriosclerosis and multiple sclerosis patients and may, in fact, be harmful.
> The health official pointed out that the manufacturer states chelation therapy does not benefit arteriosclerosis and the Federal Food and Drug Administration backs up the manufacturer's statement.

In view of this vehement opposition, it is a wonder that courageous doctors continue to administer chelation therapy.

Chapter Twelve

Professional Bias and Governmental Error in Judging EDTA Chelation

After forty years as a student and practitioner of medicine I have reluctantly concluded that much of what I have done has been a waste of time. The world is little better off and may soon be worse off than in my student days. I believe this is so because medicine — by which I mean the whole art and science of improving and preserving health, and not just that part of it performed by doctors of medicine — is on the wrong track. . . We are heading for disaster if we keep on. That is my view.
— Sam McClatchie, M.D.,
Misdirected Medicine, 1973

Modern Medicine Is Headed in the Wrong Direction

As director of the World Life Research Institute, which is an international reference center in marine biotoxicology for the World Health Organization, Bruce W. Halstead, M.D. of Colton and Loma Linda, California, was at the pinnacle of his career in 1972. Dr. Halstead, however, found himself with a serious and irreconcilable personal problem. He could not earn a living devoting himself exclusively to the investigation of the world's environmental resources and economic development. His own resources were in jeopardy. The Nixon Administration had cut off biomedical research grants and contracts that the medical scientist depended upon. Although he was then and still is a world renowned scientific researcher, an author of textbooks in toxicology, and a former medical school professor for twelve years, the scientist was lacking in sufficient financial resources to support his family. Consequently, he broadened his activities and entered the field of clinical medicine.

After extensive evaluation of basic biochemical data and clinical investigational information, Dr. Halstead began to use EDTA chelation therapy. He also adopted the program recommended by the Longevity Research Institute in Santa Monica, California.

Using these two main therapeutic regimens, the diet and chelation, and hyperbaric oxygen therapy as well, Dr. Halstead managed a dramatic reversal of hardening of the arteries for his patients. He had startling success with them. High blood pressure came down, exercise tolerance increased, and a variety of symptoms connected with the artery-narrowing process disappeared. Overall, the physician's patients thrived, and other seemingly unrelated diseases, such as diabetes and arthritis, also improved. As a result of Dr. Halstead's reduction of patients' disease symptoms, his practice grew and people flocked to his offices.

Drastically ill patients entered the physician's practice. They were people from all over the United States who had previously gone from doctor to doctor seeking some solution to their arteriosclerotic problems. Some of them had seemingly insurmountable illnesses. They were senile or had already undergone bypass surgery. In many cases surgeons had told them there was nothing more to be done. Patients arrived ready to have their legs amputated but praying that "something" could be found to save them. Diabetics came with well-established complications, such as blindness or ulcerations of the skin, and they hoped for a miracle, too. Some people were deaf because of apparent difficulties they had with excessive calcification build-up on their vestibular mechanism in the ears. Patients arrived hardly able to stand — dizzy and falling. Many already had sustained heart attacks and most knew that heart attacks were a very likely prospect. Some patients brought angiogram records that showed constricted blood vessels. The line-up of the halt, the lame, and the blind was amazing to behold.

As with other physicians who care for patients near the terminus of illness, Dr. Halstead should have been hospitalizing ten or fifteen people every day from his practice. He did not! It is a fact that although he is on the staff of three hospitals, he finds it unnecessary to admit more than one person every three months to any hospital at all. He has his patients walking, running, jogging, jumping, swimming, and going through a variety of other exercises. His patients ought to be dropping like flies that are sprayed with insecticide, but they do not. Their lives are prolonged and are given a renewed quality. Dr. Halstead's patients work at preserving themselves by using all of the different therapies he recommends.

"Yet, most physicians who chelate have to go underground with it," said Dr. Halstead. "Chelating physicians are castigated by their peers and talked about as quacks!

"Today, on the admission of the National Heart, Lung and Blood Institute of our own Department of Health, Education and Welfare, modern medicine is heading in the wrong direction," said the scientist turned clinician. "We have spent billions of dollars for the wrong research and lost millions of lives in the interval. We are faced with a plague of hardening of the arteries that literally threatens the whole of the Western world. The trend is getting progressively worse, with an annual increase in the disease of six to nine percent *each year*! Still, American medicine generally ignores chelation therapy and condemns anyone who uses it. There is something wrong with the organized arm of a profession that consistently refuses to examine the clinical and biochemical facts."

The Chelation Taboo of the San Bernardino Medical Society

Dr. Halstead told me of an incident he had with organized medicine that well illustrated his point. After being in clinical practice a few months he decided to join the county medical society and thus make affiliation with the California Medical Association. His purpose was to obtain malpractice insurance at a fifty-percent cheaper premium. "It would have been a saving of over $4,000 a year for me," he said.

His application to the San Bernardino Medical Society was held by its Credentials and Professional Review Commission, and Dr. Halstead was called to appear for an investigation.

"Well, here I am!" Dr. Halstead replied upon entering the hearing room after an exchange of amenities. "What do you want to ask me?"

The commission chairman answered, "We understand you're doing chelation therapy."

"That is correct!"

"We want to know your feeling and attitudes toward the subject of chelation therapy."

"I'm happy to give you a direct answer," said Dr. Halstead. "I have chelated in the past; I am chelating now; I will continue to chelate in the future — or until such time as I see scientific evidence that it is a totally useless procedure. Until now, I've seen nothing but very convincing clinical evidence that chelation therapy has tremendous merit for my patients. It has not been investigated thoroughly by either cardiologists or internists."

A long silence followed, with the commission members sitting and gazing fixedly at him. Dr. Halstead decided to break the silence. "Inasmuch as you have called me here to appear before a goup of my peers," he said, "I wish to explain the biochemical rationale for intravenous EDTA so that all of you will know why I have come to my conclusions about the treatment. I will go through the entire internal chelation process and describe the clinical protocol that I am following."

There were muffled sounds of grumbling from the committee members. They whispered to each other behind their hands.

The chairman replied, "This commission does not want to hear anything about the chelation treatment. We are incapable of evaluating it. And we don't really think this is the place to do it!

"Now, Dr. Halstead, this commission will conclude this meeting in about two hours, at 10:00 P.M. We will notify you then," continued the commission chairman, "as to whether your application is accepted or rejected for membership in this medical society."

The San Bernardino Medical Society seems incapable, as the chairman admitted, to judge chelation therapy, taboo or not. It has never given Dr. Halstead the courtesy of a reply to his membership application. He had applied in the spring of 1975.

The organized profession of traditional medicine, typified by that county medical society, exemplifies professional bias against chelation therapy arrived at out of ignorance. How can a group of honest physicians any place be willing to condemn almost 55 percent of our nation's population to death from hardening of the arteries without a willingness to at least look at this therapy that clearly works against the disease?

I suggest that perhaps the most deadly disease of all mankind is a mind closed to the truth, or what does not mesh with previously accepted ideas.

Medical Practice Interference by Blackballing

In the American International Hospital at Zion, Illinois, William J. Mauer, D.O., an osteopathic physician and surgeon who heads the department of preventive medicine, has been giving chelation therapy to many of his patients since January, 1976. Although the hospital staff approved the use of chelation therapy whenever a diagnosis of arteriosclerosis could be established, there is a close scrutiny by the hospital staff and the local county medical society. Hospital patients are chelated on a schedule somewhat different from medical office patients.

Dr. Mauer explained the hospital procedure during our interviews. "We perform hospital chelation in one of two ways: six days in a row and one day of rest, or five EDTA units given over a fifty-hour period with two days of rest, after which another five units can usually be given. The patients are monitored with laboratory tests such as the BUN, creatinine clearance, and twenty-four-hour urine examinations for calcium," he said.

"One of our patients, a woman with a heart problem, showed an elevated BUN test and one of the consulting physicians became concerned. He wanted to dialyze the patient."

Dialysis is the separation of smaller molecules from larger ones in kidney solutions — a method of cleaning body wastes.

"We don't have dialysis service in the American International Hospital," said Dr. Mauer, "but five miles south in Waukegan, a hospital does perform this procedure. However, my patient having received chelation therapy was not accepted to that Waukegan hospital for kidney dialysis. The hospital's physicians did not wish to become involved with a patient undergoing chelation therapy because it was different from the norm."

Dr. Mauer's experience was a blatant example of medical practice interference by blackballing. The medical community abetted by the health insurance industry seems not to mind if people die on the operating table with a nice clean cut in their chests from bypass surgery. That is accepted procedure! A heart surgery mortality rate can run as high as 50 percent. OK! But where chelation therapy is involved, professional bias or ignorance has caused patients to lose the right to life — and physicians to lose the right to give lifesaving treatment. It is practice by proscription or face boycott by one's medical peers through exclusion from use of their patient facilities and skills, even at the sacrifice of a life.

Dr. Mauer's experience was not really unusual. It is the fate of many medical pioneers, such as the Hungarian obstetrician Ignaz Philipp Semmelweis, who advised the medical establishment of his day to wash their hands before delivering a baby, to avoid transferring puerperal fever. Semmelweis was ridiculed for his recommendation and driven to insanity by his colleagues — who ignored rudimentary sanitary procedures and were known to operate while smoking cigars!

Dr. Mauer told me what happened next: "I telephoned the physician from whom I had first learned many of the chelation therapy procedures (H. Ray Evers, M.D.). He told me how to solve my present patient's problem by merely flushing out her kidneys with a little more EDTA with some extra potassium added to the infusion. That procedure worked well. However, because of the prior consultant's opinion, it was necessary that I move the woman from the American International Hospital to the Chicago Osteopathic Hospital where the renal specialist there examined her. He told me she did not require dialyzing at all. She would be fine in a few days, he said, and she was!"

Professional Bias Delays EDTA Chelation for Years

The summary of an article published in July, 1961 in *The American Journal of the Medical Sciences*, "The Long Term Use, Side Effects, and Toxicity of Disodium Ethylene Diamine Tetraacetic Acid (EDTA)," contained the statement:

> Two thousand consecutive infusions of disodium EDTA were given to 81 subjects in a study of the effectiveness of this therapy in coronary artery disease during a 2-year period. *We have found no serious side effects or toxicity with the use of disodium EDTA when administered as a 3-gm. dose and infused as a 0.5% solution over 2 ½ to 3 hours. It is, therefore, our opinion that the drug can be used without danger over prolonged periods.*
> *The most serious side effect ascribed to this agent has been nephrotoxicity, but with the administration methods described here there has been no evidence of such damage* [emphasis mine].

The authors of that article were Lawrence E. Meltzer, M.D., J. Roderick Kitchell, M.D., who was then Head of the Department of Cardiology at the Presbyterian Hospital, Philadelphia, and Florentino Palmon, Jr. M.D.[1]

Then in March 1963, *Medical World News* published an interview that quoted Dr. Kitchell as saying: "Peripheral vascular occlusive disease of the smaller blood vessels shows remarkable changes following treatment with EDTA. Candidates for below-the-knee amputations have lost their gangrene, and one ended up walking seven miles when he could not walk a block before."[2]

Dr. Meltzer was interviewed by that same medical magazine's reporter. He said, "Eleven of twelve patients with vascular disease secondary to diabetes have improved, and considering the absence of any valuable method for treating diabetic vascular disease, chelation therapy assumes great importance."[2] Dr. Meltzer expressed the additional hope that chelation treatment would avoid many of the amputations currently required because of gangrene.

One month after the *Medical World News* article was published, however, the same two authors had another article published in the *American Journal of Cardiology*. Its title was, "Treatment of Coronary Artery Disease with EDTA — A Reappraisal."[3] Amazingly, these two research physicians who had for years been writing articles that sang the praises of EDTA chelation, suddenly pulled a giant reversal on the therapy. Even as the medical news reporter was interviewing them, the physicians had a directly opposite viewpoint in the press. It was a superficially negative article — the only negative one published on the subject — which had a devastating effect on the entire therapeutic concept of EDTA chelation. That 1963 "reappraisal" article changed all orthodox medical thinking about the therapy, so much so that it has yet to recover from the effect.

Busy clinicians, it seems, relied on the conclusion of this negative 1963 article by Kitchell and Meltzer. Until now, traditional physicians have not taken the time to carefully read every word in the article. Such a careful reading would have strongly suggested the conclusion was not statistically valid. They would have learned that "below the knee" artery circulation was improved, for instance. Doctors need to reevaluate chelation therapy in light of all the new developments in the field. Then they would learn that the Kitchell and Meltzer article's significance is totally neutralized by a comprehensive review of the literature. This literature includes publication of at least twenty clinical articles about the benefit of EDTA in vascular disease in particular and another 1,700 articles on the general subject of chelation for other medical uses. Additionally, there are about 6,000 science articles published describing the chelation action in nature.

Garry F. Gordon, M.D. explained to me the events that occurred after publication of the Kitchell-Meltzer "reappraisal." Dr. Gordon said, "The negative reappraisal by Kitchell and Meltzer virtually stopped all chelation progress in this country for twelve years. Yet, I have recently talked to Dr. Meltzer on the telephone for hours, and he has admitted to me that he had been pressured extensively by National Blue Cross and Blue Shield to come out against chelation. He told me confidentially over the phone during 1976 that he believes chelation therapy may be the most beneficial of treatments known to mankind, but until we can tell our medical colleagues exactly how it is working we should not broadly promote it.

"And as for Kitchell," Dr. Gordon continued emphatically, "his last published work,[4] two years later, in 1965, still cites the beneficial results of chelation in vascular disease and diabetes, and he has never published again. I ask you — or anyone — is the negative reappraisal valid at all? Kitchell has published no other article. His total scientific writing before his

EDTA assertions were several articles supporting the use of internal mammary ligation which turned out to be only a placebo effect."

The internal mammary artery ligation for alleviation of angina pectoris has been abandoned by chest surgeons. This operation was shown to provide only a "wished-for" effect — an imagined effect — on patients.

"One day I will blow this whole 'reappraisal' article on chelation wide open! It calls for some very astute investigative reporting of the most fascinating kind," Dr. Gordon said.

"Funding for the Kitchell and Meltzer EDTA research was from the John A. Hartford Research Foundation. The Foundation gave them $1,000,000, and they ostensibly set out to attempt to duplicate the clinical results of Dr. Norman E. Clarke [5,6] that he had published in 1956 and 1960. When the anticipated clinical improvement did not occur immediately after treatment, Kitchell and Meltzer were almost ready to abandon the project.[7] Then research was continued because their review of the protocol required reevaluation of the patients after three months, otherwise the researchers might have lost their grant-in-aid. Surprising to Kitchell and Meltzer, they found the angina of their patients was much improved — on the order of 90 percent. They therefore went ahead with further investigation," said the AAMP past president.

"A co-author with Drs. Kitchell and Meltzer on chelation research was Marvin J. Seven, M.D.," Dr. Gordon continued. "He was a brilliant researcher who, unfortunately, committed suicide at age thirty-one in 1961 during the period of the Kitchell and Meltzer research and publications on chelation. His death virtually terminated any major interest in chelation treatment for several years. Dr. Seven had devoted great energy to the development of EDTA chelation therapy and helped arrange the first two major symposiums on chelation which were held in 1959 and 1960.[8,9] Those symposiums were attended by scientists and clinicians from many of the leading medical centers and research facilities throughout the United States, including such research centers as Stanford University, Brookhaven National Laboratories, Cardiovascular Research Laboratories, Baltimore City Hospital, the California School of Medicine, the Dow Chemical Company, and many others."

Dr. Gordon showed me a textbook edited by Marvin Seven called *Metal Binding in Medicine*.[8] It contained the entire proceedings of the first symposium. Apparently, owing to Dr. Seven's death, the second chelation symposium, held in September 1960, which he had helped to organize, did not appear as a published book. Rather it is listed in the medical library in the form of a periodical entitled: "Proceedings of a Conference on Biological Aspects of Metal Binding."[9] The series of such setbacks help to explain the uphill battle for chelation, until now.

At these two symposiums on "metal binding" and EDTA chelation, scientists of multiple disciplines sat down together and exchanged information.

They agreed that during the ten years since EDTA had been introduced in this country fantastic therapeutic results were already being recorded. Clinicians talked to pharmacologists and to biochemists. That year, 1960, many exciting reports about the therapeutic effects of EDTA chelation therapy were presented, but the journal that carried this important information never came to the attention of the general medical community.

Then, as now, almost half of all deaths were related to hardening of the arteries. The field of chelation therapy was just beginning to attract general medical interest around the world and was starting to take hold in the United States. But Marvin J. Seven, M.D., the young and dynamic leader who was sparking the chelation therapy movement, killed himself. The people who looked upon his work with admiration asked, Why? There was speculation of all kinds. But no one in the United States moved to carry on Dr. Seven's work and, therefore, it was left for investigators in other countries to develop further the chelation concept. Clearly beneficial results in arteriosclerosis have been reported in Germany, Russia, and Czechoslovakia. [10,11,12] The agent is employed to reverse hardening of the arteries in those countries. And those foreign physicians give full credit in their references to the early American physicians who discovered this use of EDTA.

The Erroneous National Research Council Report

The combined efforts of Drs. Seven, Kitchell, Meltzer, *et al* have had far-reaching effects on the lives and pocketbooks of us all. In general, physicians themselves never have read the complete articles, but they have responded to the few article excerpts reported in medical journals and textbooks. Most of these have focused on seemingly negative comments contained in the one article labeled "A Reappraisal." Even government agencies prefer this one negative article. The U.S. Government has issued statements based on a clearly erroneous report predicated on the Kitchell, *et al* research paper, particularly their reappraisal. [3]

This 1963 article was picked up and the five other plainly positive studies performed by those authors were ignored. Government agencies concentrated on the negative aspects, which in reality were really *neutral* conclusions in the article. The medical bureaucrats failed to acknowledge the openly favorable aspects contained in the same report!

The Panel on Cardiovascular Drugs of the National Research Council of the National Academy of Sciences was asked to consider the use of Endrate (EDTA) in vascular occlusive disorders. The FDA made that request and a report resulted. This vital report was written to record, once and for all, the erroneous work of Kitchell and Meltzer. But several major errors were made in the report!

In one error, the NRC mistakenly attributes a negative conclusion to the researchers' 1960 paper, when that particular publication was extremely positive. The authors had been highly impressed with the potential of chelation treatment, and clearly stated so, although their haphazard and inadequate testing methods could well have resulted in total failure. That original 1960 study reported on ten patients who were initially disabled with severe persistent angina pectoris. The patients' conditions could not be controlled by other known therapies at that time, so they were treated with disodium EDTA. The bare adequacy of Kitchell and Meltzer's treatment programs caused essentially no improvement to be noted by either patients or investigators after the first series of treatments, [13] and they planned to abandon the experiment, as Dr. Gordon has described.

The doctors had not counted, however, on one of the most important characteristics of the chelation treatment. The loss of pathologic calcium and removal of cholesterol and other fatty debris from the interior arterial walls apparently continues long after the conclusion of a course of EDTA therapy. Reports of improvement began coming back from the chelated patients, and the doctors reevaluated all ten of them three months after they had completed their initial series of chelation treatments.

Unforeseen by the researchers, three months after the beginning of their experiment, nine of the ten patients were showing reduced frequency and severity of anginal attacks. They had a reduced requirement for nitroglycerine. They had increased their exercise tolerance. Of the nine who originally had abnormal electrocardiograms, five now showed improved ECGs. Most impressive of all, the three patients who had first indicated enlarged heart size when viewed by X-ray now showed reduced heart size. The investigators declared these positive results a direct effect of the EDTA chelation. This was exactly as Dr. Clarke had described in his 1956 article! This positive response caused Kitchell, *et al* to continue their chelation research on more patients, none of whom were ever given nutritional therapy or a program of exercises. In short, the patients did not change their lifestyles. Thus, even though chelation gave good symptomatic relief to many patients, it did not seem to significantly extend the life expectancy of those who were treated, simply because the patients continued with their atherosclerotic way of life.

Then the 1963 "Reappraisal" hit! [3] No one has been able to explain the turnabout on any logical basis, and the authors kept contradicting themselves. They ran a foolishly designed study that anyone can read about in that second article. A medical scientist will immediately see the inadequacies of its design. Kitchell and Meltzer failed to establish an adequate or comprehensive therapy. Instead, they attempted to treat a polygenic (an interaction from many variations) with only one active therapeutic agent that actually increased the chances for complications from arteriosclerosis to later occur. How? Because of the mineral deficiencies they knew they induced — but did not treat. The two researchers also tried a double-blind cross-over investigation which was doomed to failure, and they arrived at conclusions that were not at all justified by the data.

Most ridiculous of all, Kitchell and Meltzer said the chelation therapeutic effects were "not lasting." But consider this: diabetics who would quickly die without their daily injections of insulin have been known to live full and vigorous lives for decades, and nobody criticizes insulin injections because they are *not lasting*. Why then do Kitchell and Meltzer condemn intravenous injections of EDTA on that basis as "not a useful clinical tool"? A conclusion like that for insulin would be recognized as idiocy, and it is idiotic to say the same for EDTA. This is particularly true since zinc and chromium are recognized as involved in arteriosclerosis. As a physician, you would not leave patients deficient in these essential trace minerals and expect their EDTA injections to keep them alive and free of past disease. That would be stupid, and medically negligent as well.

The National Research Council Makes Its Awful Error

A reportedly responsible quasi-governmental agency that supposedly checks its facts first, the National Research Council (NRC) has accepted such illogical conclusions despite five other positive reports from the same authors. The NRC has made an awful mistake by this silly acceptance and created additional havoc in the bargain. It is an error that cannot readily be forgiven by the families and friends of those who have died from being denied EDTA chelation because of publication of the NRC report. Everyone in the United States, directly or indirectly, relied on that NRC report — but it was not checked for accuracy and, in addition, the error was compounded and made worse.

Another error, one that shows outright dishonesty or utter indolence, is that the NRC purports to quote verbatim from the Kitchell and Meltzer positive paper of 1960 when it, in fact, actually must have been quoting from their 1963 reappraisal article. Then, *they erroneously claimed that both studies were negative.* [13] The National Research Council's Medical Consultants and bureaucrats obviously did not read that 1960 paper all the way through. Certainly they did not quote from it verbatim. It is incredible to realize that actually there are five reports favorable and one somewhat unfavorable which were written by these authors, as I have pointed out, and the NRC report concludes all of their studies are negative. In my research of the literature, uncovering this tragic error had me in shock. It indicates the height of laxity by scientists in the highest seats of office.

A third error is the NRC statement that says, "Investigations by other authors are little more than testimonials." *Frustration* is another word that best describes this medical journalist's feeling, when I hold in my hands twenty additional, plainly valid, published studies by other clinical investigators.

Why has the National Research Council selected the flawed, inadequate, self-contradictory, and illogical writing of the single Kitchell and Meltzer 1963 "Reappraisal" paper? Such a selection reminds one that, prior to the

Wright brothers' flight at Kitty Hawk, expert scientists examined the failures and supported the dictum that man would never be able to build a machine that could fly. Even to this day, the NRC report leads the Federal Government and the medical establishment to insist on remaining earthbound by shackling themselves down with oversight, stubbornness, and error. Thus the patients who would want chelation therapy — and their physicians who would offer it — apparently must be deprived of a most effective anti-atherosclerosis treatment because they do not know what it is, or they think its benefits will not endure.

We, the people, are the big losers by this completely incorrect NRC report. It shades the opinion of any doctor who would use it as a legitimate reference on EDTA chelation. Any medical researcher or clinician who relies on its erroneous finding will receive a seriously distorted picture. Worse still, the effects of this wrong NRC report continue to this day. For example, Medicare continues to refuse to pay for chelation, citing a 1969 decision that relies on this faulty NRC report.

A near-final note: If, in fact, Kitchell and Meltzer had found negative results initially, which had stayed negative throughout their studies regarding the effectiveness of chelation treatment, that would have been a solid case against the therapy. Rather, Kitchell and Meltzer co-authored five articles before the 1963 one, which favorably discussed chelation therapy. Still the unexplainable professional bias as manifested by their "reappraisal" article, combined with the awful governmental errors, have set back the use of chelation therapy in the United States for years. It seems obvious to me that Kitchell and Meltzer were pressured into a change of heart.

Chapter Thirteen

Government Harassment of a Chelating Physician

Sometime ago I suggested in a memo that it was not fanciful to suspect that the ethics which we saw at work during the Watergate affair had not been confined to politics. . . We know from our own experience in Washington that high federal officials countenanced dubious behavior as regards our work. . . . It is unlikely that so important an activity as science can be apolitical: apart from anything else its politics impinge upon it so heavily, that it is the duty of scientists to insure that its morals and ethics are not eroded.

> — A memo from Humphrey Osmond, M.B., M.R.C.P., F.R.C. Phych. to Abram Hoffer. Ph.D., M.D., F.A.O.P., F.R.C.P. (C), March 27, 1975

Eugene Carlson Avoids Triple Coronary Bypass

"The first signs of my heart trouble started in the summer of 1975," said Eugene Carlson, an automobile mechanic of McKeesport, Pennsylvania. I spoke with Mr. Carlson after I arrived in Pittsburgh on January 21, 1977 to attend a meeting of the National Health Federation. Mr. and Mrs. Carlson were among the audience attendees who were anticipating the appearance of H. Ray Evers, M.D. of Montgomery, Alabama, the scheduled speaker. I too expected to listen to that famous chelator and then interview Dr. Evers for this book. This physician, one of chelation therapy's foremost pioneers, never did arrive to address that meeting, because he was being watched day and night by the U.S. Government. Agents were waiting for Dr. Evers to make some medical mistake — anything at all — so they could take away his professional license, get him sued, put him in jail, or worse. They have attempted all these things already. I will tell you the whole story about the man's experiences shortly.

In the meantime, Mr. Carlson agreed to be interviewed, as a substitute for the missing speaker. He described how EDTA chelation had eliminated the need for his having to undergo a triple coronary artery bypass operation. Mr. Carlson's medical tale took on rather dramatic form, as do most of these experiences connected with chelation therapy. Those who come to use the treatment often do so as a last resort, when it should be their *first* resort.

"I got short of breath while cutting grass one day. I just did not seem to have the energy to do the daily and weekend jobs around the house that I had always done," Carlson told me. "I let the chores go more and more. During the winter, shoveling snow in a cold wind bothered me very much, too. After a while, I felt a crawling sensation along the chest that did not go away, and I became even more short of breath. Then I felt pains in my left arm.

"In April 1976, I went to my family doctor to have a complete physical examination. The doctor said that my blood pressure, triglycerides, and cholesterol readings were very high and my heart was skipping every third beat. He gave me blood pressure and heart pills and made an appointment for me to see a cardiac specialist in Pittsburgh.

"The specialist put me in St. Francis Hospital in May for a heart catheriza-tion [an arteriogram]. When he read the results, this heart surgeon said I needed three or four coronary artery bypasses. 'But Gene,' he said, 'I might get you on the operating table, cut you open, and sew you right up again without doing much of anything because there would be too much occlu-sion.' I realized then that I really was a sick man and I sure needed help," Carlson said.

While talking to me Carlson shook his head from side to side and beads of perspiration formed on his forehead as he recalled the doctor's diagnosis. Mrs. Carlson stood nearby and shook her head also, in confirmation. He said that he thought seriously about accepting the risks of open heart surgery, even though the operation might net him nothing.

"I was talking to my dentist about my possible chances of coming out alive from the operation," Carlson said. "He told me of his friend, Max Weiss of White Oak, Pennsylvania, who had gone through a similar problem but solved it by going to Belle Chasse, Louisiana for chelation treatment. I didn't know where the place was or what the treatment was.

"I visited Mr. Weiss over at White Oak and talked to him. He described his experience and referred me to others who had gone through the treatment. I talked to many of the people that he mentioned. They included Nick Jurich and many of the folks who have attended tonight's National Health Federa-tion meeting," Carlson pointed out. "After that, I felt I'd rather chance the medical treatment with chelation than undergo any heart operation."

Mrs. Carlson recalled the tension-filled weeks they lived through. She said that they spent many anxiety-ridden nights talking over the prospects of Eugene's life-or-death situation.

Carlson said, "I called Dr. Evers and told him of my problem and asked if he thought he could help. He made no claims of curing, but he said he felt that chelation would help my arteries get cleaned out and then with the aid of the correct nutritional program such as diet, vitamins and minerals, I could keep myself in much better health."

Smiling broadly, Carlson said, "He has been so right. I feel better today than I have in a long time. The only worktime I lost was while I stayed in the Meadowbrook Hospital in Belle Chasse. Then I took off just two more weeks after I got home. I do a lot of vigorous work on my job in the garage.

"I went to my family physician in December 1976 and had myself checked again. My blood pressure, triglycerides, cholesterol, and electrocardiogram readings were all very good — normal, the doctor said. And my heart no longer skips a beat. I had taken treatment from Dr. Evers in July 1976. I took twenty-five chelations then. After the first week at his hospital I quit taking the heart pills that I brought from home, and to this day I haven't needed them. I know I'll never have to take heart medicine again — that's how well I feel."

The Big Worry Always in the Forefront

Eugene Carlson has one worry though — that Dr. Evers, or any other physician in this country, may not be allowed to continue giving EDTA chelation. Mr. Carlson's alarm came sharply into focus while he was a patient at Dr. Evers' Meadowbrook Hospital. During his stay, he and his fellow patients felt compelled to circulate petitions that asked the State of Louisiana and the U.S. Government to stop the harassment of Dr. Evers. The patients asked the authorities to remove the pressure they were putting on the hosptial staff and to keep open the hospital's doors. (The hospital was about to be forced to stop its activities. In fact, it was shut down soon after Carlson had his treatment.)

In an effort to stop Dr. Evers from using EDTA for treatment of circulatory diseases, on two occasions in 1975 the FDA designated his chelation drugs as misbranded and seized them. This was totally without precedent, as the FDA had always insisted that it had no control over the private practice of medicine. Nevertheless, government officials marched into the hospital supply room and removed the bottles of synthetic amino acid solution from its shelves. The FDA had gotten a court order permitting it to do that.

In my later talk with Dr. Evers, he said: "The judge said that I had misbranded the article for arteriosclerosis and used it for treatment of this disease, which is not listed on the drug insert. Therefore, the judge said, I misbranded it because it was shipped in interstate commerce."

As I described earlier, I was present at the Pittsburgh meeting Dr. Evers was to address. In an open line telephone conversation broadcast to the audience, he explained that this very evening the FDA and the Alabama State Licensing Board of Medical Examiners were watching him closely at his newly relocated clinic in Montgomery, Alabama.

The Remarkable Medical Wanderings of H. Ray Evers, M.D.

H. Ray Evers, M.D., a Southern gentleman and Presbyterian Sunday

School teacher, learned about EDTA chelation in 1965 from the late Carlos P. Lamar, M.D. of Miami, Florida. The two physicians gained national reputations among those familiar with chelation therapy. They developed large medical practices. Some 400 physicians scattered throughout the country took their chelation training from Dr. Evers. Approximately 1000 practicing physicians today actively use chelation therapy in some form. Dr. Evers is known now as the treatment's most prominent living exponent. The 66-year-old physician has given chelation treatment to over 16,000 patients.

The Columbia General Hospital of Andalusia, where Dr. Evers began to practice chelation therapy in 1965, had a sixty-bed capacity which he had built from his general practice income. Treatment with EDTA infusions then started to expand tremendously. People began arriving daily from all over the United States. They wanted to avoid dying of hardening of the arteries or becoming part of the 10 or 12 percent (or more!) patients who died attempting bypass surgery.

The chelating doctor needed more beds to accommodate the large number of patients for whom he had no room. They clamored for him to save their lives, their limbs, or their loved ones. The word spread throughout Alabama, and sick people arrived with or without appointments to receive this mysterious treatment that they had heard created "miracles." This Southern country doctor rose to the demand; he expanded the hospital. Still, more people kept coming to Andalusia, a sleepy little town in the deep South.

Having a lot of land, Dr. Evers just continued to build on new hospital wings and hire more staff. He increased his hospital's capacity to 160 beds. Then the physician discovered that he had been earning too much money too fast. He developed a Federal tax problem. The hospital bookkeeping records had been sorely neglected, because Dr. Evers was kept busy as the medical director, hospital administrator, nursing supervisor, purchasing agent, and other duties all rolled into one. With financial records such a terrible mess, he hired a certified public accountant to correct things.

The tax matters were finally straightened out. His accountant recommended that the best thing Dr. Evers could do was to purchase an insurance policy that would pay him a million dollars when he was sixty years old and to donate the whole hospital with its land, equipment, medical supplies, and various sundries to the Presbyterian church as a tax write-off. He followed the accountant's advice and gave the hospital to the church in which he taught Sunday school. Dr. Evers' office remained located within the hospital.

As the years passed, the patients kept arriving in droves. They came from foreign countries as well as from around the United States. The church elders, the physician's old cronies who were the Columbia General Hospital's Board of Directors, began to drop off the board, one by one. Either they died or moved away or were replaced with alternate members.

Up to then, he had taken no notice of his loss of board control. But suddenly one day Dr. Evers found himself facing an entirely new hospital board. They handed down uncomfortable new restrictions. First the board members charged him office rent, where there had been none before. Then they levied telephone charges for his intercommunication to the hospital. The Board of Directors realized that if something happened to Dr. Evers, their hospital would be in trouble, since 75 percent of all its patients belonged to him. It was usual for the chelating physician to have ninety people hospitalized at one time. He was too powerful, the board believed; the hospital could use some other medical leadership, said the murmurings.

This new board heard in hysterical language how new physician leaders on the Board of Directors described chelation treatment as unethical and unorthodox. "The hospital will get sued," they were warned. "Just think of the bad publicity. Evers isn't practicing traditional medicine like everyone else. It's out of the medical mainstream! Chelation treatment isn't even mentioned in medical school! It's poisonous, dangerous, murderous! How can we be a party to murder?"

The hospital board agreed to pass a resolution that said as of February 1st of the following year there could be no more chelation therapy given at Columbia General Hospital. Dr. Evers was told to cease chelation treatment at once and dispense orthodox medical care, or prepare to leave the hospital — the hospital he personally had started!

In January, as the Board's anti-chelation deadline approached, Dr. Evers arranged to take up medical practice and accept hospital priviliges in Atlanta, Georgia. The Atlanta Eye Hospital, owned and administered by one of his physician friends, offered to rent him an empty wing. Dr. Evers moved like a whirlwind to transfer all of his patients by ambulance and airplane to the new facility. He had acquired a temporary license in Georgia. He practically emptied the Columbia General Hospital of all of its patients.

Dr. Evers Moves Again

A falling out soon developed between Dr. Evers and the Atlanta Eye Hospital owner. They were, unluckily, two very strong-minded and stubborn men who differed about how much the Alabamian should pay the Georgian to buy the facility.

Dr. Evers then accepted another invitation, one offered by the Seventh Day Adventists. They invited the physician to use their new twenty-million-dollar facility in the Georgia capital. The Atlanta West Hospital had multiple floors, one of which was offered entirely for his use to administer whatever treatment he deemed necessary. Dr. Evers could conveniently have his personal office on the same floor. Again he moved his patients.

The Atlanta operation ran smoothly for a short time, until spite and jealousy broke through the dignified veneer of other medical professionals. Envy consumed some as they saw the accommodations and consideration given to the new physician. Several doctors complained that their recently arrived hospital colleague had not applied for staff privileges through the usual channels. Collectively, doctors and nurses charged bias in Dr. Evers' favor. The staff asked for a meeting to air their complaints openly, and Dr. Evers was not allowed to attend.

A clause in his contract gave the Atlanta West Hospital's Board of Trustees the singular right to rule on Dr. Evers' staff privileges. His patients had been moved to the Atlanta West Hospital, in part because he would not need to go through the rigmarole invariably involved with gaining hospital staff privileges. Besides, the Alabamian lacked the time to wait for rules, regulations and protocol connected with a big city hospital. Still, staff members sided against him and refused to acknowledge the unusual circumstances of his arrival.

The entire medical staff began a boycott of their 450-bed hospital. General services were reduced. Patients were left largely unattended. The media picked up the story and ran with it for many days. Pressure built on Dr. Evers from all quarters. Finally, he was forced to withdraw from the Atlanta West Hospital and from the State of Georgia as a whole.

Big City Publicity Hits a Little Louisiana Town

The physician concluded that to conduct his hospital practice successfully he must control administrative policy. Consequently, Dr. Evers began to search for a facility that he could buy outright. He finally found one reasonably priced in Belle Chasse, Louisiana, a town of 13,500 population outside of New Orleans. Even before the physician held a permanent license to practice medicine in the State of Louisiana, he took possession of the Meadowbrook Hospital.

What do you think is going to happen when a small, dusty, antebellum sort of Southern town, slumbering in non-activity, suddenly is swamped by people from the North and other places, who are looking for Lourdes-like cures against sickness and death?

Referred patients from far and near descended on the unprepared Belle Chasse populace. Each desperate and disabled person was ready to hang up crutches, wheel chairs, sacks of medicines and other impedimenta of invalids on the town walls. It was a medical nightmare — a sociological bane to the once somnambulant community.

The town folk of Belle Chasse experienced culture shock similar to the citizens of Plains, Georgia, when Jimmy Carter first became President of the United States. Churches were shaken by the schism. Local politics was polarized. Taxes increased along with the appreciation of real estate. And day after day, week after week, scores of cars with out-of-town tags rolled slowly into town looking for the Meadowbrook Hospital. Coincidental with the arrival of patients, news reporters and feature writers descended on the town. The press gave the rural community more publicity than it wanted.

A Belle Chasse Patient's Story

Joseph Gaudio, a forty-seven-year-old bachelor from Palm Desert, California was one of those patients who spoke to the press. "I am grateful beyond words. I was directed by God to go there," he said, for what he believed was a life-saving treatment.

A treadmill test and angiocardiogram taken at Eisenhower Medical Center in California indicated that without heart surgery Mr. Gaudio might have but two more years to live. Two of his major coronary arteries were 95-percent clogged with fatty plaque, and a third major artery was 70-percent blocked.

Gaudio explained that at Cedars of Lebanon Hospital in Los Angeles, a heart specialist told him "I'd die in two years if I didn't have the surgery, a three-way bypass . . . my appointment was with a doctor in Pacific Palisades who . . . told me that statistically, the surgery was 'not all it's made out to be in the long range' — they don't get at the cause," said Gaudio.

"I asked him what the alternatives were and he said, 'None. I wouldn't make any long-term investments, you're sitting on a powder keg, you could go any moment,' " the former patient repeated.

Then Joe Gaudio learned about Dr. Evers from Betty Lee Morales, a contributing editor of *Let's Live* magazine. He telephoned the physician to learn about the treatment given, and he rechecked with three other physicians because the patient was fearful of "quackery." While the chelation theory "seemed to make sense" he still was undecided, he said. The three doctors told him, "if chelation were any good, we would be using it."

After six more telephone calls to Dr. Evers in Louisiana and weeks of indecision — "mental torture, believe me!" — Gaudio finally boarded a plane for Belle Chasse. He remained at Meadowbrook Hospital from August 6 to September 28, 1974, staying two more weeks than was considered necessary because, he said, "I wanted to be sure everything was okay." The treatment made him feel like a new person because of a resurgence of energy he experienced — "something I hadn't had for years. Bang! I felt like a million dollars!"

Some time after his return from Meadowbrook Hospital, Gaudio arranged to take a treadmill test at Loma Linda Community Hospital. He did not reveal his history to the medical intern there. The usual stress test exercise was given with the stress set at 173 heartbeats per minute. "I hit 170, and he told me there was no indication of any problem. I asked if he would let me run on it for a bit; he said it wasn't necessary, but agreed since I was persistent. He set the stress at the starting point, and I ran for ninety seconds, reading a stress point of 175. I couldn't have done that last year," said Joseph Gaudio.[1]

Many other dramatic testimonials like Gaudio's were ballyhooed around Louisiana, and this sort of publicity turned neighboring physicians against Dr. Evers. Additionally, some people in surrounding communities left their physicians or transferred themselves out of hometown hospitals and into Meadowbrook Hospital. Local physicians did not care for that very much, either.

Attack from the Louisiana Medical Board

Roman law was the basis of legal procedures in Louisiana under both the French and Spanish regimes. After admission to the Union in 1812, the state made many attempts to establish a legal basis similar to that of the other states. The result has been the development of a legal system that rests on the French and Spanish codes in the area of civil law and largely on English legal precedents in criminal law.[2] As a result, it is remarkably easy to become licensed to practice medicine or most other professions in the State of Louisiana.

Using his credentials from medical school and reciprocity from licensure in other states, Dr. Evers had been granted a temporary license to practice medicine until the Louisiana Board of Medical Examiners met again in three months. Then he was sure to receive a permanent license. He had accepted his three-month permit and leased the Meadowbrook Hospital in Belle Chasse with the privilege to buy. I understand that Dr. Evers took possession of the facility even before the temporary license came through.

A growing backlog of patients were literally camped on the hospital's doorstep waiting for Dr. Evers to take possession. Some had very little time left to live. They begged for treatment. A few of the ones who were viable, and could undergo heart or artery surgery, probably did so during the physician's practice hiatus from Atlanta to Belle Chasse. Others who wished to become his patients may have died while they waited for the hospital to open.

From investigations I have done to uncover facts about H. Ray Evers, M.D., one major criticism is accepted even by his fellow chelating physicians. They say that he lacks the ability to say no. He won't tell a hopeless victim, "I won't give you chelation treatment because your physical condition is beyond hope."

Dr. Evers gives care to whoever feels they need it. Even recognizing that a person is just days away from death, he will tell the patient's family confidentially, "The condition is impossible and past hope, but I'll try to do something anyway." Humanitarian reasons aside, that is medical misjudgment, his colleagues say. Dr. Evers counters with "remember the oath of Hippocrates!" But the professional criticism has been leveled and has validity in the minds of his critics, friends and admiring colleagues though they may be.

As a result of this physician's attitude over the years, some of the most severe cases of hardening of the arteries in the whole country — perhaps in the world — have come under Dr. Evers' care. Patients have been brought to him who were critically close to death. A few thousand people have had their lives saved and health restored, but a few dozen others, indeed, have died just as predicted.

Several physicians, even fellow AAMP members with whom I spoke, fault him for recognizing but not accepting patient risk factors that were obviously too great. They shake their heads and say almost in unison, "Dr. Evers has put himself and chelation therapy in jeopardy. He has taken any patient who crawled to his door. That's taking too hazardous a risk with one's reputation and with the validity of the treatment. Why doesn't he consider the rest of us who are chelating physicians? Sometimes we have to defend the therapy because of patients about to die but given chelation treatment anyway. Look at the heart and artery bypass surgeons! They operate only on those patients who are the healthiest. They won't accept just *anyone* for heart surgery. The vascular surgeons make sure to keep their mortality statistics as low as they possibly can."

When several cases — without hope but treated by Dr. Evers anyway — did die, the news was picked up by the New Orleans television stations. Histrionic human interest stories broke in the newspapers nationally about patient deaths. Some were wire services stories. One news story I found in the *Salt Lake Tribune* for August 22, 1976 reads: "The FDA reported ten deaths at the hospital associated with chelation agents as well as several patients who required dialysis . . ."[3] What the various national news reports neglected to mention was that in most cases these people died from terminal cancer, *not* from any side effects of chelation therapy. The therapy had been given by Dr. Evers in response to pleadings by family members as a last resort, to hold a little longer to the thread of a loved one's life. But as a consequence of the news stories, when the Louisiana Board of Medical Examiners met to consider making Dr. Evers' license permanent, his request was denied. The medical examiners predicated their decision strictly on the press reports of these ten deaths with which he was connected.

Louisiana Troubles Had Just Begun for H. Ray Evers

Being denied a permanent Louisiana medical license was just the start of more legal and governmental troubles for Ray Evers. Here was a physician in possession of a hospital, with hundreds of patients pounding at its doors to get in, yet he remained without a license for a year. In the meantime, Dr. Evers hired John R. Potter, M.D. to be his Chief of Staff at the hospital. Dr. Evers took on the role of hospital administrator, which did not require a medical license.

On January 14, 1976, he filed a new motion for permission to present additional evidence to the medical examiners. This was granted, and the Board held a hearing. Witnesses flew in from various parts of the country in support of Dr. Evers. Joseph Gaudio was one of a hundred patients who offered to testify in the physician's behalf, and he was granted the privilege.

"Dr. Evers brought my 'before and after' reports to the hearing — those from California showing the condition I was in when I went to Meadow-brook, and then the treadmill and circulation report from Meadowbrook. About eight doctors were at the hearing. [Five of them sat on the Board of Medical Examiners.] One asked how I felt," said Mr. Gaudio, "and I told him 'great' — like a nineteen-year-old. I thought of course they would examine the reports on my case, but no — they didn't bother to look at them."

The Board again denied Dr. Evers a license to practice medicine in the State of Louisiana, and obtained a temporary restraining order against him as well. They declared him incompetent. And, because he charged for treatment, they accused him of defrauding the public as well. The chairman of the board openly stated that he would see that Dr. Evers never got a Louisiana medical license.

As he had for the previous year, Dr. Evers continued to permit chelation therapy to be administered at his hospital despite the restraining order. He was subsequently arrested. The Medical Board of Examiners had made its move. He was sentenced to ten days in jail on a contempt charge. Later the sentence was voided by the Appeals Court.

While the matter of Dr. Evers' license remained on appeal, a group of patients and friends joined together and formed the National Educational Society for Natural Healing, 1717 Homer Street, Metairie, Louisiana 70005. Under the leadership of Fred J. Doughty-Beck, D.C., this group won a civil class action suit June 20, 1975. Under its new president, Herbert Stahl, Sr., the National Educational Society for Natural Healing has since expanded its membership to thirty-seven states. The class action suit that it won caused the Parish Court to issue an order to enjoin the Louisiana State Medical Board of Examiners from depriving Dr. Evers of his license to practice. As we shall soon see, however, this was only a temporary victory.

Meadowbrook Hospital Also Under Attack

To stay out of jail on further conviction of contempt, Dr. Evers avoided all direct patient care and acted strictly as administrator of Meadowbrook Hospital. His skills and talents of more than thirty-eight years were totally denied to patients. Medical services were rendered by a staff of qualified professionals under Dr. Potter's medical direction.

Then, Meadowbrook Hospital also came under attack. Its license renewal was delayed by the State Board on Hospitals. The excuse given was that it had no surgical department, which was true. This institution specialized in preventive medicine and the medical care of degenerative diseases. It referred patients for surgery to other institutions when absolutely necessary. Dr. Evers' attorney, Kirkpatrick W. Dilling, filed for a hospital review hearing.

A grand jury hearing subpoenaed all of Dr. Evers' hospital records on two separate occasions, without doing anything with them except to make copies. Record keeping, in truth, is another critical fault of Dr. Evers, as friendly fellow physicians had told me. They admit he is notoriously weak in this record-writing area.

"He doesn't document well enough," one of his supporters said. "Several of our AAMP (American Academy of Medical Preventics) members have gone very deeply into this inadequate documentation with him. In most ways Evers is far ahead of other physicians in practicing preventive medicine — except in documenting what he does in practice. There he remains just a country doctor." Dr. Evers admitted the same thing to me, himself.

The grand jury looked over Dr. Evers' records as a prelude to possibly filing criminal-civil charges against him. Although his record keeping no doubt could have used much improvement then, there was nothing in Dr. Evers' actions that were criminal or negligent. He received a clean, impartial ruling, and the grand jury ended its interest.

Inadequate documentation of case histories was a minor weapon used by both Medicare and Blue Cross to blitzkrieg Meadowbrook Hospital. Their major complaints also were that the hospital lacked twenty-four-hour operating room service and did not do major surgery. They joined together in a decision not to pay any of the hospital's charges to patients. These two main hospital insurance coverages in the United States were denied to that institution. Thus, patients received no hospital benefits. Chelation care was not covered, patients were told, and either they paid the hospital charges out of their own pockets when they expected the bills to be paid by health insurance, or the hospital did not get paid at all.

A Federal Appeals Council had ruled, you may recall from Chapter Nine, that such payments must be made, as in the December 1, 1975 decision of J. J. Dominey, Sr. But Medicare and Blue Cross have carried that issue further. Each case must be adjudicated on its own merits by a series of suits and appeals. Few patients will take the time or spend the legal fees involved. In fact, even Alabama Blue Cross and Medicare still owe Dr. Evers a large amount of money from his practice in Andalusia, Alabama, years before.

Persecution by the FDA and IRS

The Federal Food and Drug Administration, in an entirely unprecedented action, entered the anti-chelation attack on Dr. Evers, as I have mentioned previously. The FDA seized the Meadowbrook Hospital's inventory of disodium edetate on grounds it was misbranded. The governmental agency charged, "EDTA labeling not only carries no recommendations for its use in circulatory disease (*USA vs DISO-Tate*, DC La) but even states that 'chelation therapy is contraindicated in generalized arteriosclerosis associated with aging' [circulatory problems]."

Dr. Evers counter-attacked with a civil rights action in Federal Court. A patients' civil class action was filed in Louisiana's Plaquemines Parish Court asking for a restraining order. An injunction was issued against the FDA. The physician's counter-charge stated that this FDA action was a vicious invasion of the rights of a physician to prescribe medication for patients. But the bureaucrats still were not through with him. Then the Internal Revenue Service stepped in.

The IRS Charges Evers with a Felony

Dr. Evers was behind in paying his 1974 income tax. A penalty and a fine were assessed on him by the Internal Revenue Service. By May 1976, he had scraped together $25,000 and paid the back taxes, with just the penalty and fine remaining.

About two weeks after his tax payment, an IRS officer arrived at the office door of Dr. Evers to impound his automobile. The IRS agent had no bill of charges and gave no prior warning. He demanded the car, he said, because the government wanted the automobile as collateral for approximately $2500 still owed by the physician.

Dr. Evers was enraged and used strong language in reply. He explained that the tax principal was paid and the penalty and fine soon would be paid. Meanwhile he was paying the government its usual interest. The IRS agent still wanted his car keys. Dr. Evers shouted that the IRS' demand for his car was illegal, since a doctor's vehicle is a tool of his trade, needed to make house calls and to get to and from the hospital. He refused to give up his car. The IRS agent finally left.

In response, however, the government tried to indict him for a felony, claiming that he attempted to run down the IRS agent. If a physician had such a conviction, it is probable that he never would be able to acquire or retain a medical license anywhere in the United States. In that way the IRS was offering a sister governmental agency, the FDA, a little extra assistance. Luckily, no indictment could be made to stick. There was a lot of legal hassling and warding off the police in between, though.

Dr. Potter and the Meadowbrook Hospital staff went on obtaining and administering EDTA to patients with arteriosclerosis. Again the FDA took legal recourse. It obtained its own unprecedented injunction ordering the hospital to stop stocking the chelation drug. The requested injunction was granted on grounds that without such restraints the government agency would be forced to resort to daily seizures to enforce the removal of the "misbranded" drugs from interstate commerce. The injunction also required notification to patients that the hospital was forbidden to hold or use the drugs.

Then the State Medical Board of Louisiana induced the Orleans medical parish to badger and put under pressure Meadowbrook Hospital's chief medical officer. John R. Potter, M.D. had been there as a member of the staff since the hospital opened in 1974. He was the licensed Louisiana physician that ran Meadowbrook, but because of horrendous vilification he experienced from fellow physicians and the medical examining board, he finally was harassed into resigning. Dr. Evers had no licensed physician supervisor to take legal responsibility for patients.

Dr. Evers Abandons the Louisiana Fight

During the FDA trial in the summer of 1975 in New Orleans, the FDA attorney, Guy Pffifer from Washington, D.C., admitted before Judge Gordon that Dr. Evers was being singled out for individual prosecution and destruction. It was said that if the Federal Government could prevent him from practicing medicine, any other physician who attempted to employ EDTA chelation therapy could be shown Dr. Evers as an example of the consequences of such a misdeed. He was, after all, the chief teacher and leading proponent for the intravenous treatment. "Get Evers and you'll stop them all," was the word circulating in the Department of Health, Education and Welfare.

In twenty-six months of legal battles, Dr. Evers spent $142,000 in legal fees. He remained without a license to practice medicine in the State of Louisiana and could furnish no other licensed physician on the hospital staff. He was warned, "If you are caught even taking a person's blood pressure, you will be put in jail for a year and receive a stiff fine."

Bureaucrats told him to get out of town within thirty days or be hit with the next harrassment. He closed his hospital and left Louisiana when news came to him that other governmental agencies were ready to move in.

Dr. Evers Moves to Montgomery, Alabama

Dr. Evers next leased a forty-bed clinic in which he offered chelation therapy in a new technical form — The Ra-Mar Clinic in Montgomery, Alabama. The FDA followed Dr. Evers to Montgomery and filed a suit, civil action 78-93-N (*United States of America vs. H. Ray Evers, M.D.*) in the United States District Court for the Middle District of Alabama, Northern Division. The FDA tried to stop him from doing chelation therapy of any kind — not just with EDTA. In June, 1978, it filed for an injunction for him to "cease and desist." It was a test case for every physician in America. If Dr. Evers had lost the case, the judgment against him would have affected the medical practice of every U.S. doctor. He or she would have lost the right to deviate in any way from the instructions on the package insert of a drug.

"No doctor could give penicillin for an abscess tooth because the package insert doesn't recommend penicillin for this purpose," explained Dr. Evers. "The judge asked the FDA lawyer, 'You mean if I went out and played golf and sprained my ankle and I called my doctor, the doctor couldn't suggest I take aspirin because it's not recommended for ankle sprain?' "That's correct your honor," said the lawyer.

"I had two hundred witnesses — patients — at court ready to testify about what was done for them. The judge heard ten of them testify in my behalf.

The time was getting lengthy, and the judge turned to the FDA lawyer and asked, 'Will you stipulate that these other one hundred and ninety witnesses will tell similar stories? If you don't we'll be sitting here a whole week just listening to them.' Some of the witnesses were other lawyers, physicians, and one was a Supreme Court judge from the State of North Carolina. They finally came to an agreement to stipulate that the whole two hundred witnesses would say something beneficial in my behalf," said Dr. Evers.

United States District Judge Robert H. Varner ruled that the government, or anyone else, has no right to determine how a physician must practice. "The FDA in trying to get an injunction for chelating of any kind would have stopped me from using aspirin, penicillin, or other drugs because they all act by the process of chelation," Dr. Evers pointed out. "However, the judge ruled that I was doing nothing wrong and as a doctor I had the right to choose the method of treatment. No one could interfere with my right to practice medicine. This ruling protected the medical practice rights of every physician in the United States."

There is still harassment, of course, and Dr. Evers has been driven to seek a haven away from official and quasi-official interference. Dr. Evers has moved his clinic facilities once again, and has opened a new medical plant for the practice of chelation therapy in the Bahamas. He has begun taking patients at Whale Point Retreat, Harbour Island, Eleuthera, Bahamas.

Chelation therapy is still under the gun in the United States. A not-so-subtle conspiracy seems to be afoot in the land. Led by a variety of special interests, mostly in conflict with the needs of the medical consumer, it has reached into the agencies of government. More doctors who use ethylene diamine tetraacetic acid (EDTA) in the treatment of arteriosclerosis are being tracked down and oppressed by commercial and political interests. The treatment has practically been made illegal except for human elimination of another mineral poisoning — lead rather than calcium. Don't you wonder why? If it is recommended by the Department of Health, Education and Welfare in the lead detoxification of children, why cannot EDTA chelation be used to prolong the lives of adults that are young, old, healthy, sick, enthusiastically alive, or on the threshold of death? In the next chapter, I shall present you with some answers to this puzzle.

Chapter Fourteen

The Conspiracy Against Chelation Therapy

For the sick and diseased, the restoration of health is the overriding concern of their lives. For the healthy, the threat of illness and disease, while less immediate, remains a "brooding omnipresence." While good health and the absence of disease is always a central private concern, it is only in the last few decades that it has emerged as a central public concern. Yet two hundred years ago we pledged our society to safeguarding "life, liberty and the pursuit of happiness." Is there any human condition which more directly and poignantly denies to us those inalienable rights than dread disease and inadequate health care? A government which does not direct its energies to the eradication of disease or injury and does not provide its citizens with basic health care is as derelict as that government was from which we declared our independence almost 200 years ago.
— U.S. Senator Warren G. Magnuson,
How Much For Health, 1974

A Conspiracy that Could Kill

A former violinist with the Cleveland orchestra, Bert Arenson of Cleveland, Ohio, underwent double coronary artery bypass surgery in late spring, 1973. The operation was only partially effective. In less than a year Mr. Arenson experienced coronary insufficiency almost as severe as before the procedure. He quickly realized that his health situation was absolutely unendurable.

Arenson found himself unable even to stand for more than five minutes without angina. Pain pierced his chest with any exertion. Walking for the man was confined to his home — going from room to room — slowly and infrequently. In fact, any effort led to irregular heart rhythm and immediate chest discomfort. He could not tolerate cold temperatures; even stepping out of his house brought on heart symptoms. "My whole problem was getting worse and deteriorating rapidly. It became quite clear — I did not have too much longer to live," Arenson said.

His cardiac condition made reconsideration of further bypass surgery seem foolish. The patient had blockages downstream from his vein-artery grafts, in the small arteries beyond the bypassed main branches. Surgery could not reach them, and except from EDTA chelation, there is at present no effective threatment for this occlusive arteriolar condition in the heart. After the obvious failure of the first operation, the cardiac patient could foresee no benefit from additional open heart surgery.

Fortunately, Arenson watched a television documentary on chelation therapy. He became curious, but held his enthusiasm in check until he could learn more. His wife Sylvia investigated this potentially life-saving treatment. She made long distance telephone inquiries, studied clinical journals at the medical library, and spoke with people about the procedure. The therapy was then unavailable in their home city of Cleveland or in any of the nearby states. Within a month Sylvia embarked with her husband for Miami, Florida, so he could receive chelation from Carlos P. Lamar, M.D.

By the end of six months of travel back and forth to Miami and forty-five EDTA infusions, Arenson was walking briskly two and a half miles daily, even in freezing weather, which ordinarily is not possible for angina patients.

Half a year later, the heart patient had finally located a Pittsburgh physician who would administer the therapy. But he was struck down by acute cardiac insufficiency and was hospitalized the evening before he was to begin another course of chelation. The appointment came too late to prevent his latest heart seizure.

His emergency cardiologist at the Pittsburgh hospital held out no hope that the man would get better following his heart attack.

"The picture was terribly gloomy," Bert Arenson told me. "But then the hospital authorities allowed something unprecedented and really unusual. They permitted me to travel by ambulance daily to the office of Howard T. Lewis, Jr., M.D. of Pittsburgh for five days of chelation therapy during my second week in the hospital."

Improvement of the patient was so obvious and rapid that in a few days the hospital's doctors and nurses and even the cleaning women looked at him in wonderment. His skin color changed from sallow to normal, appetite returned, and he could walk without feeling chest pain or gasping for a breath, as he did before the chelation. Arenson left the hospital and continued with twenty more infusions which he received from Dr. Lewis.

Since that time of cardiac crisis, the patient has taken additional chelations regularly. He has now received a total of 148 treatments. Now they are administered to him by a family practitioner in Cleveland, James P. Frackelton, M.D., who recently became interested in providing this treatment.

The Conspiracy Against Chelation Therapy

Some powerful, established institutions feel threatened by EDTA chelation therapy. They are the driving force behind an unspoken, unacknowledged, but powerful movement to illegitamize disodium-EDTA treatment. They want chelation therapy eliminated from the American scene. Even now, only a few courageous physicians have the temerity to use disodium ethylene diamine tetraacetic acid (EDTA) in their clinical practices.

Why is *anyone* against intravenous EDTA? Why do certain special-interest groups fight so hard against the treatment being made generally available? Why are there, in fact, vested interests cooperating in a conspiracy against the therapy? Who are the conspirators? What do they have to gain? I know the answers to these questions and, by the time you have completed reading this chapter, you will know them, too. Then perhaps together we can begin actions that will force our government to permit us to use this basic health care to reverse hardening of the arteries.

Four powerful interest groups are apparently conspiring to keep chelation therapy away from the American people. One group has evolved from the collective efforts of vascular surgeons, heart surgeons, chest surgeons, anesthesiologists, the administrators of hospitals with bypass surgical facilities, cardiologists, internists, other physicians, and self-serving politicians from the American Medical Association. These specialized groups collectively claim that the EDTA chelating agent is dangerous and unproven. They point to the lack of double-blind research studies. Yet, these same physicians permit and even encourage *more dangerous and unproven* bypass surgery to go on, with a known ten-percent mortality rate.

HEW's two intradepartmental agencies, the Social Security Administration and the Food and Drug Administration, support each other to form a second special interest group. These Health, Education and Welfare agencies are aided by sister governmental departments and make up an intragovernmental collusion. Their cooperation is in direct violation of our constitutional rights as private citizens.

Pharmaceutical companies combine to prevent EDTA from coming on the market, and they comprise a third conspiring group. Theirs is a kind of economic boycott, which is markedly unfair to the medical consumer in its effect. This counter consumer attitude is motivated by a few factors which I shall describe, but all of them are tied to money.

The health insurance industry is committed, as much as possible, to preventing health insurance policy holders from being reimbursed for chelation treatment. They seem to fear that although eventually it would save them much money which today is wasted on surgery, too many people would take the treatment who now take nothing to prevent or reverse hardening of the arteries. Or perhaps they are simply responding to pressure put on them by the medical and political establishments. For whatever reason, the health insurance companies act as a fourth conspiratorial group to block the acceptance and widespread use of chelation therapy.

The American Medical Conspirators

As it becomes more widespread, the effects of chelation therapy on the American medical profession, particularly the specialists of internal medicine, cardiology, heart surgery, chest surgery, vascular surgery, and anesthesiology, will certainly be devastating. Fewer patients will seek out these medical professionals to receive their services. The high prices they have been commanding will have to drop precipitously. Expensive equipment will go unused. A tremendous reduction in the utilization of hospital operating rooms, hospital beds, nursing homes, and medical clinics will be another result.

I have said that cardiovascular disease is the largest single cause of disability and death in the United States. My statement is supported by the American Heart Association, which estimates that heart disease alone presently costs the American public more than fifty billion dollars a year. And the AHA projects that the figure will go much higher.

As an industry, the sale of medical services for just cardiovascular disease is not far behind the automobile industry. American medical traditionalists are not known to waste all of their built-up hospital facilities and the investments they have made in bypass surgical equipment. Certain highly trained specialists are not going to sacrifice their cardiac surgical skills to become just good samaritans and exist on the five to ten percent of patients who may still have some form of vasculary surgery performed after they have received chelation therapy. The loss of various securities and endowments would be too great. [1-3]

Something is quite wrong with the present orthodox medical system that requires more and more bypass surgical patients to keep expensive equipment operating. An excess of catheter-trained cardiologists are disgorged into the health ranks each year. There is an overabundance of cardiovascular surgeons. [4] The shift from primary-care physician to specialist has caused an excessive use of invasive cardiologic techniques. [5] Our country has become overly oriented toward vascular surgery. Still, the medical investments have been made and organized medicine is attempting to make these investments pay off.

Administration of chelation therapy does not require the supervision of a medical specialist. No extra technical training is required. The approximately one thousand doctors now providing EDTA infusion around the United States are mostly general practitioners, who often are less vulnerable to the constraints imposed by medical specialty boards than the specialist. The treatment is usually given in a physician's office with extremely effective results. General practitioners soon discover that they hardly need to refer their patients to other medical specialists at all. And they seldom require hospital facilties for their patients.

EDTA chelation is highly effective — simply too effective — for the medical profession. That is the reason disciplinary actions in obvious open restraint of trade are being taken against chelating physicians.

Medical Pressure Against Another Chelating Physician
The case of Robert J. Rogers, M.D. of Melbourne, Florida is typical of how

organized medicine is attempting to thwart the use of chelation therapy. He is a physician I described in Chapter One. In November, 1975, the Brevard County Medical Society expelled Dr. Rogers and ordered him to stop giving chelation treatment, which he had used since 1970.

The medical society held a hearing on Dr. Rogers after Dorothy M. Shamp, of Port Angeles, Washington, wrote to complain, saying her mother had received EDTA chelation from the physician in 1974. Mrs. Shamp said that over a three-month period her mother, Ruth Norris, spent between $1,500 and $2,000 for treatments and examinations — "nearly half of the equity she received from the sale of her home."[6, 7] Dr. Rogers' records, however, show that Mrs. Norris paid $884 for all treatments and examinations over a six-month period in 1974.

Mrs. Shamp admitted in a January 1977 telephone interview that while her mother praised the treatments, she, Mrs. Shamp, was suspicious of them simply because she had never before heard of chelation.

At the medical society hearing Dr. Rogers was not allowed to present objective medical evidence, such as the tests on his patients, which proved the effectiveness of the treatment. Nor were his patients permitted to testify about the benefits they had received, or that chelation was *their* preferred treatment.

Since Dr. Rogers would not agree to stop using chelation, he was expelled from the Brevard County Medical Society, which also brought the matter to the attention of the Florida State Board of Medical Examiners. Dr. Rogers' license to practice medicine in the state was in jeopardy.

His hearing before the state board was held in Orlando, Florida, September 10, 1976. He was represented by Attorney Andrew Graham, who raised serious legal questions, including one regarding the qualifications of the board's medical witness, Waldo Fisher, M.D., a medical researcher at the University of Florida who disputed Dr. Rogers' claims for chelation. Dr. Fisher is not an "expert" on chelation, as he has no professional expertise with EDTA or chelation therapy, said Attorney Graham.

Despite this, the board gave the previously written recommendation of Robert C. Palmer, M.D. of Pensacola, Florida full ratification. Dr. Palmer represented the Brevard County Medical Society. He wrote, after hearing testimony from Dr. Fisher and Dr. Rogers, "The use of such method of treatment by a private practitioner in a manner that must be categorized as haphazard and flippant . . . fails to conform to the standards of acceptable and prevailing medical practice."

The Florida Board of Examiners ruled January 21, 1977 that Dr. Rogers be put on one-year probation, with the stipulation that his license be revoked if he continued to use chelation therapy.

With assistance from the American Academy of Medical Preventics, Dr. Rogers filed an appeal against the Florida Board of Medical Examiners' order with the District Court of Appeal, First District State of Florida. The case (R.

1324-1326) took two years and the expenditure of about $20,000 by the physician. Furthermore, the board's action had an adverse effect on his practice, of which only twenty percent involved chelation. In conversations with Dr. Rogers, he told me, "People were reticent to come to me for care. It cost me considerable in time, money and distress."

Then, January 11, 1979 a three-judge panel ruled strongly against the medical board — both the Florida Board of Medical Examiners and the Brevard County Medical Society had their actions criticized. Acting Judge Tyrie A. Boyer in the First District Court of Appeal ruled the medical board had no authority to deprive a doctor's patients from therapy they want, unless it can prove "unlawfulness, harm, fraud, coercion or misrepresentation."

Just because most of the medical profession rejects a certain method of treatment, the court ruled, does not give the state medical board authority to punish a doctor for using it. Then, in a moment of philosophical musing, Judge Boyer wrote, "History teaches us that virtually all progress in science and medicine has been accomplished as a result of the courageous efforts of those members of the profession willing to pursue their theories in the face of tremendous odds despite the criticism of fellow practitioners." He compared Dr. Rogers to Copernicus, Pasteur and Freud as an innovator in science and medicine. He said those scientists were first ridiculed and then lionized for their unorthodox ideas. But how many other physicians in Florida, witnessing such persecution of a fellow M.D. by his peers, would have the courage and convictions of Dr. Rogers? How many were cowed into silence — and ignorance — about chelation by the medical establishment?

Anti-Chelation Conspiracy by the Federal Government

In collusive action, the Food and Drug Administration helps the Social Security Administration avoid payment of Medicare claims. I alluded to this collusion in the last chapter. Here is how it is done: Anyone who writes for information about EDTA chelation therapy to HEW — this includes Fair Hearing Officers, Social Security Appeals Council adjudicants, physicians representing medical peer review committees, state boards of medical examiners, attorneys, private citizens, and other correspondents — receives a standard diversionary letter from Peter Frommer, M.D., Associate Director for Cardiology, Division of Heart and Vascular Diseases, National Heart and Lung Institute.

Bert Arenson of Cleveland received that standard letter designed to sidetrack inquiry, but he refused to accept it and invoked the "Freedom of Information and Privacy Act" to acquire 360 pages of FDA documents that make up its anti-chelation file. Copies of Dr. Frommer's standard letter and other form letters are among the documents. They had been used many times.

Dr. Frommer's standard letter is an inaccurate "model" response that has been sent out to the public for about the last six years. The words have not varied, and his inaccuracy prevails. This, despite five cartons full of clinical articles, patient records, studies, diagnostic tests, charts, graphs, recordings and other supporting proofs of therapeutic benefit afforded by chelation treatment delivered to FDA headquarters in July 1974 by Harold W. Harper, M.D., who at that time was president of the AAMP.

Also, Dr. Frommer continues to mail his incorrect letter in the face of increasing information available through the National Library of Medicine Literature search #70-36.

On careful review of Dr. Frommer's documents, we learn that if he thinks you are an opponent of chelation therapy or a proponent in disguise, it is important enough to him to put a "memo-to-file" in the FDA file to identify clearly your stance. He sends a different letter to a chelation opponent than the letter he sends to a proponent. The opponent's letter clearly demonstrates the FDA's awareness of important substantiating clinical research articles which his "standard" chelation proponent's letter seems to deny exist. In other words, if he thinks you're pro-chelation, his letter tends to discredit the therapy. If he judges your stand to be against it, he tells you some of the truths about what it's able to do therapeutically.

A typical collusive event was revealed in a file letter of August 11, 1969 entitled: "MEETING TO REVIEW INTRA-HEW VIEWS ON EDTA." In this letter, it is clear that Dr. Theodore Bedwell, Chief Medical Officer, Bureau of Health Insurance, Social Security Administration, wants some guidelines established for Medicare reimbursement policy. Evidently Dr. Bedwell already knows that the decision will be against payment for chelation therapy, as he introduces this conclusion himself in his letter.

This policy to deny payment for chelation therapy for patients under Medicare has resulted in thousands of claim denials. As we know from Chapter Nine, a dozen or more patients with these claim denials have made the effort to demand so-called Medicare "Fair Hearings," and have collected some money under Part A. Nevertheless, Medicare, Part B claims are continuing to be denied reimbursement, based in part on queries by Fair Hearing officers to the Bureau of Health Insurance (Dr. Bedwell's department) and the DHVD-NHLI (Dr. Frommer's department). FDA-Social Security System collusion effectively avoids payout to the elderly for life-prolonging chelation treatment.

Does the Social Security Administration WANT Us to Die Sooner?

The Social Security System is not self-funding, and the Social Security Administration has so bungled its mandate that you and I are working today to pay into the System to support citizens who retired yesterday. The more retirees who live to ripe old ages and the longer they live, the more money it will take for the Social Security System to support them.

Currently, 22,789,000 people at age sixty-five exclusively, others at age sixty-two, plus younger citizens who have been disabled, 35 million people in all, receive about thirty-one percent of their prior average monthly wage, or about $291.77 per person per month, as benefits to live on. This amounts to $3,501.24 a year on which the beneficiary pays no income taxes. Considering only those age sixty-five and older, we see that the Social Security Administration thus pays out approximately $80 billion in annual benefits to maintain just its 65-year-old retirees.

The cost would really be critically burdensome if all of us increased our life expectancies. Suppose we live an average of just one more year. That being the case, our nearly 23 million Social Security recipients age 65 suddenly would cost the Social Security Administration another $80 billion each year. Indeed, the cost would escalate far beyond that dollar figure, because of the bell-shaped curve that develops because people live two, three and even five years longer than average. Could the United States afford to have its population live an extra year? The entire annual budget for this nation in 1979 was about $496.2 billion. The retired elderly would, therefore, require an additional $160 billion.

In other words, if millions of Americans suddenly discovered a procedure that would enable them to live longer, healthier, happier lives, it could bankrupt the federal government. There is simply not enough money to pay the increased Social Security benefits that would be required. The clear implication is that the Social Security Administration would prefer us to die sooner and not later. Otherwise financial demands would soar far beyond the system's ability to pay.

Chelation therapy administered to those older people who need it is a big potential source of that extra financial burden. Social Security Administration career bureaucrats in authority know this. They know if just one retired recipient's case is reimbursed by Part B, Medicare, the next recipient will deserve payment, and the next. The bureaucrats fight tooth and nail to avoid reimbursement for chelation treatment bills. Remember the story in Chapter Nine — how they fought the D. D. Dominey case? They still refuse to accept that case as a precedent for Medicare, Part A chelation bill payment to hospitals. They require each case to be judged on its merits and thus fought through the "Fair Hearing" officer and possibly on to the courts.

I have mentioned in several earlier chapters that all of us suffer from hardening of the arteries to some degree. The longer you live in general, the narrower your arteries grow. For nearly 23 million arteriosclerotic retired elderly, taking chelation therapy at an average individual cost of $2,000, the total treatment cost to Medicare would be $46 billion. This medical cost could come on suddenly like an erupting volcano. Informed people will want it quickly to enhance the quality of their lives. All kinds of diagnostic services would also be involved.

The average individual $2,000 medical fee for chelation therapy includes laboratory and physical tests before chelation, the treatment itself, tests afterward, medicinal or food supplements for the patient, and follow-up of the patient by the physician for at least three months afterward. It is understandable, albeit not ethical or humane, that HEW intradepartmental agencies support each other against Americans living longer. They attempt to block us from taking EDTA chelation treatment for their own valid financial reasons. Only, the Department of Health, Education, and Welfare has been created to work for our benefit and not to our disadvantage. Some changes in policy have to be made.

The Criminal Oversight of the FDA

As a sister agency of the Social Security Administration, the Food and Drug Administration carries out HEW's present penurious policies with disdain for the public's requirements. It would deny Americans the right to elect the use of this or other essentially non-toxic therapy for themselves. The agency allows us no freedom of choice, even if patients wish to pay for that choice. The FDA and other governmental agencies expend money and energy in attempts to suppress the availability of EDTA chelation.

When the Kefauver-Harrison Act was passed in 1962, EDTA chelation therapy was clearly accepted as the "treatment of choice" for arteriosclerosis by experts who were knowledgeable in this particular area. Then the error was committed by the National Research Council, which I reported to you in Chapter Twelve. The error significantly impeded widespread acceptance, or even any further investigation, of EDTA chelation in the United States. Reviewers working with the NRC to evaluate EDTA in cardiovascular disease for the FDA clearly misinterpreted the Drs. Kitchell and Meltzer literature. They erroneously reported that "both" of their published clinical studies were negative. This erroneous report remains the NRC official position today — despite the AAMP's attempts to bring the error to the FDA's attention. Allowing such an error to remain amounts to criminal oversight, but it is not entirely without precedent.

In fact, the AAMP has been denied any FDA hearing at all. The Academy responded to the *Federal Register*, volume 39, #137: July 16, 1974, which stated that any person who desired a hearing should file a written notice to request such a hearing by August 15, 1974. AAMP did so. That is when Harold W. Harper, M.D. took a trip from Los Angeles to the FDA headquarters in Washington, D.C. with five file boxes of supporting material.

J. Richard Crout, M.D., Director of the Bureau of Drugs, Department of Health, Education and Welfare, spoke to Dr. Harper for twenty minutes, after which he referred the then AAMP president to a group of several physicians in his department. These physicians said that the FDA *only* accepted research data from drug companies and *not from private practicing physicians*. Thus all of the volumes of material delivered to them demonstrating "before and after" testing of patients' circulatory status with thermography, plethysmography, EKGs and computer analyses of the degree of symptom relief following chelation therapy, were utterly ignored then, and they continue to be ignored to this time. So-called responsible government officials remain uninformed regarding the overwhelming documentation existing in the literature in support of the treatment. The FDA still holds those AAMP documents, but they disregard them to this day. This also is a criminal oversight.

These problems with the FDA and NRC were reported to the head of the Subcommittee on Oversight and Investigations of the House of Representatives, Representative John Moss of California, in a lengthy letter dated January 7, 1977 by Garry F. Gordon, M.D. To date, *no* response of any kind had been received to his letter requesting assistance. One must wonder why Representative Moss ignored the public's need. Enough public outcry against this suppression may force other congressmen to act on behalf of the American people.

Additionally, no correspondence has ever followed that complete turndown by Dr. Crout's representatives. Since then, nonetheless, there has been a continual harassment of chelating physicians by the FDA. The agency persists in collusive efforts to suppress chelation therapy in our country. As I have described, it seized a supply of EDTA from H. Ray Evers, M.D. and took unprecedented legal action by going into court against him. The FDA claimed that Dr. Evers' use of EDTA involved the "misbranding of EDTA," whereas they previously sent him a letter dated March 7, 1974 clearly stating that the use of a legally obtained drug in the doctor's office is "the practice of medicine" and is not within their jurisdiction.

The FDA has harassed drug suppliers who have been told that since EDTA is not cleared for use in arteriosclerosis, they must limit their sales of this substance to 100 bottles per month. The FDA has no clear right to take this action, particularly in view of the agency's failure to grant the full hearing regarding EDTA requested by AAMP in 1974.

Curiously, EDTA was originally developed, and approved as safe and effective by the FDA, for treatment of relatively minor conditions. Moreover, some 90 million pounds of the substance were produced and used in the United States last year, much of it as preservatives in our foods. We all get it one way or another, but not the *right* way: intravenously, where it can do some good.

A physician is legally permitted to use any "approved" drug for any purpose, according to his own judgment. Yet, even while ignoring existing legal precedent, the FDA continues in its attempt to dictate the practice of medicine and backs up its attempts with drug seizure. The agency sometimes uses its multi-million dollar annual budget and its thousands of staff members seemingly against the best interests of the American people.

Pharmaceutical Companies Are Another Conspiring Group

EDTA, used for intravenous injection, has been in the public domain for a long time. I previously pointed out that its patents had expired and, unfortunately, there is no real profit for most pharmaceutical companies in making and distributing it. They are therefore not willing to invest any money in EDTA to prove through research its use in preventing or reversing hardening of the arteries.

The pharmaceutical companies may not want to disseminate general information about EDTA, even if they could, because the substance's latent potential is to compete for sales with their current, fully invested, and highly profitable drug products. These products number in the thousands and include such items as drugs for hypertension and angina, vasodilators for arteriosclerosis, and others for problems resulting from impaired blood circulation. Intravenous EDTA therapy might eliminate the need for all of them.

To adequately document the therapeutic effects of EDTA on hardening of the arteries, a really large and rather expensive study has to be undertaken. To satisfy the purists in science, the study theoretically should be a double-blind controlled investigation that would cost millions of dollars. A pharmaceutical company with faith in its patented product ordinarily underwrites this sort of study. Understandably, with no clear-cut patent to protect its financial interests, no pharmaceutical company is going to foot the bill for an extensive double-blind investigation, even though the government offers some "label protection" on drugs which can no longer be patented. Pharmaceutical industry executives are not altruists. They are business people, often with stockholders to report to, and they must have a return from investment.

But the pharmaceutical industry can be severely faulted as a group conspiring against chelation therapy in another way. A few years ago the pharmaceutical package insert that described the effects of EDTA injection listed calcified arterial disease as a viable use (that is, "possibly effective"). That listing has now been removed. Melting under the heat of FDA demands, Abbott Laboratories and other EDTA manufacturers have taken a negative step away from preserving the nation's life and health. By agreeing to the removal of the indication for occlusive vascular disease from the package insert, the pharmaceutical companies have, in effect, affirmed their own disapproval of the use of EDTA chelation for hardening of the arteries. This action has left physicians with a previous warning against use of the drug in "generalized arteriosclerosis associated with aging" to explain to their potential or actual medical malpractice claimants. That statement made some sense when above it the package insert recommended the product in angina and other blood vessel conditions. Now without those possible indications the chelating physicians have an additional legal obstacle in using EDTA for their patients. Even the FDA is unable to come up with an explanation why the negative statement about its use in arteriosclerosis prevails. Why was it put there in the first place? No one offers an answer.

On its own, the AAMP researched how to get EDTA moved from "possibly effective" to "proven effective" for purposes of FDA regulations. The FDA referred AAMP officers and directors to Abbott Laboratories, which had already done the basic new drug application on EDTA many years before. AAMP contacted Abbott Laboratories for assistance in completing the necessary paperwork for its application. The AAMP physicians proposed that they would append their physician-sponsored investigational new drug application to Abbott's basic NDA. This procedure would incorporate the data the physicians had accumulated on EDTA to make a meaningful application for FDA purposes. It would be no extra trouble for the pharmaceutical company.

To finance the additional research they intended, and to do it without help from the pharmaceutical industry or the U.S. Government, all the AAMP physicians assessed themselves $600 each. Suddenly, in response to pressure from representatives of organized medicine who are chelation opponents, Abbott Laboratories cut off the friendly relationship it had developed with AAMP members. Perhaps Abbott did that as protection against FDA or organized medicine reprisals. Without Abbott's cooperation, the executive committee of AAMP decided to temporarily postpone the research project on EDTA and vascular disease which the physicians had planned to accomplish. Then the AAMP physicians found they had to spend their research funds to fight organized medicine to maintain their physician rights to offer EDTA treatment to their own patients. The battle is being fought now. The research funds set aside by AAMP must be wasted in defense of those doctors to practice medicine in the way they know best will help their patients.

We Need Double-Blind Studies

HEW's chief spokesman on chelation, Dr. Peter Frommer, demands that double-blind studies be performed to prove chelation therapy is a low-risk therapeutic procedure. But no one will do them — and the medical establishment and political bureaucracy stop anyone who wishes to try. Clearly, it is time these studies be carried out, under federal or private foundation sponsorship, with funds allocated for full-blown medical research of EDTA.

Yet bypass surgery is done daily in the United States without the "appropriate controls" asked for by Dr. Frommer of EDTA chelation physicians. Studies were done in the evaluation of the Mammary Artery Ligation Operation, and it was determined that this surgical procedure, quite popular in the 1960s, was apparently primarily producing a "placebo effect." In other instances, some double-blind studies attempted in psychiatry have also shown serious deficiencies with this form of medical care.

Some chelation opponents feel that the EDTA infusion therapy may be a placebo. They are certainly welcome to that opinion. Nonetheless, as long as eighty percent of chelating physicians' patients stop having angina and leg cramps, recover their memories, do not need any amputation of gangrenous legs and toes, and find vision returning, it should be considered a useful therapy, placebo effect or not. Currently, none of the chelated patients die as a result of this safe, effective, non-surgical approach.

The pharmaceutical industry, as I have noted, has a tremendous investment in cardiovascular and ancillary drugs. But it must also invest in drug advertising to get any single product sold. No pharmaceutical firm is going to spend additional millions of dollars to clear EDTA through the FDA for cardiovascular disease and then more millions to promote the drug. Why? The reason is that they could not protect their investment. Anyone can make EDTA. Other drug companies would get a free ride. They could make and sell the same substance, although they might not be allowed to state the same claims on the package insert for a period of time. In the meantime, the investing company might never recover its costs.

Promotion for a drug is necessary in American medicine. No practicing physician adhering to the AMA line would have the temerity to use any drug not heavily promoted in medical journals by the drug industry. A physician puts his career on the line recommending *any* treatment other than the usual, reasonable, and customary one. Drugs promoted in medical journals are considered usual, reasonable, and customary. The drug companies are forced to spend many millions in drug promotion; otherwise, a physician will refuse to use the non-promoted product.

The Role of Health Insurance Companies in the Conspiracy

I have pointed out that widespread use of alternative cardiovascular therapies will have a considerable effect on medical practice. There is now no generally effective treatment for patients who suffer from vascular occlusive disease. The medical profession's response has been to provide little treatment other than to simply observe the course of the patient's arteries as they are undergoing their hardening. When the patient's condition becomes severe, either he dies or he becomes a candidate for vascular surgery. Simply put, in most cases the non-holistic-type orthodox practice abandons the patient. Palliative segmental surgery is sometimes carried out — for a disease that is not at all segmental. Vascular surgeons may attempt to repair your heart or your legs, but arteries in your head still remain diseased. And this medical neglect is aided and abetted in a not-so-subtle manner by the health insurance industry.

Health insurance companies refuse to deal with treatment of a person's entire arterial system. Their health insurance policy payout is biased, instead, in favor of crisis-oriented medicine. Health insurance is like fire insurance. The house has to catch fire before a fire insurance company will pay on its policy. The same goes for your health — or loss of it. "Health" insurance should be called "sickness" insurance, since you must be sick before you can receive reimbursement on your policy. The only way you or I can collect third party compensation is to undergo some emergency or crisis medical care, such as surgical bypass. Diseases must be well established before there is any financial assistance from our carrier. We receive no preventive treatment, or very little, that is reimbursed by health insurance.

We do not even get compensation for comprehensive medical checkups because we feel some chest pain. With no diagnosis, there is no reimbursement. In other words, the health insurance industry pays us to be sick and ignores us if we remain well. It is the ultimate in negative living — reimbursement only if we get sick.

If chelation therapy were to become an accepted modality, it soon would be widespread in use. The net result might be an upset in the immediate financial balance of many insurance carriers. Long term savings through the diminished need for intensive-care procedures, high-priced surgery, prolonged hospitalization, and other medical expenses are not being projected by them. Insurance executives seem to see only the initial costs of treating a possible 115 million potentially arteriosclerotic patients among our populace in the first few years that chelation therapy becomes popularly accepted. They don't want to pay for this sort of preventive medicine.

Yes, it is clear that preventive care may cost more initially. But the long-term savings to the carriers could be tremendous, if only the new diagnostic methods were put to use in a concentrated preventive medical program. The procedures already exist. New sensitive tests, such as treadmill cardiology, noninvasive laboratory techniques, plethysmography, systolic ejection times, high-speed retinal vessel photography, omnicardiography, Doppler ultrasound, hair analysis, and early stroke-risk detection with thermography, have come into more common use. These techniques, instruments, and machines diagnose disease processes at an earlier stage.

Thus, more and more patients who now receive only watchful observation as treatment could request or receive EDTA chelation. This would let them live longer without disability. Costs to insurance carriers for health maintenance of policy holders might be formidable at first. Insurance company executives certainly recognize this. Some patients who know of chelation treatment have accepted bypass surgery of the arteries, simply because it was covered by their insurance policies and EDTA chelation therapy was not.

The health insurance companies' opposition to chelation therapy comes down finally to that secret motivating word — *money*. Even though chelation treatments for policy holders represent significant long-range financial savings to the insurance carriers, they opt instead for crisis medicine and emergency intervention. Actuaries have shown insurance executives that with continued encouragement for the practice of crisis medicine only a few patients survive to reach major medical centers where they receive very expensive medical care. Or, many patients refuse surgery, preferring to let events take their natural course instead. The health insurance companies can thus get off the hook early in a cardiovascular patient's illness. He soon dies!

Immediate implementation of a program of EDTA intravenous treatment to potentially 115 million policyholders at a cost of $1,500 to $2,000 each would possibly bankrupt all the health insurance companies several times over — up to $230 billion worth! Obviously, that seems to be a present fear of carriers. Of course, this would not happen in one year but the payout might occur over a ten-to-fifteen-year period. People would live a lot longer and be a lot healthier.

The evil tentacles of the health insurance industry conspiracy reach into every chelating physician's practice. The importance of insurance carrier reimbursement to a physician's patients for the financial well-being of a professional practice is clear. Patients rely on their health insurance to pay for the majority of major medical expenses. Many patients who do not get paid are forced to limit the medical services they seek or go elsewhere for their care. Chelation therapy is sacrificed, and its preventive approach cannot be instituted. Crisis medicine then must continue as an individual patient's ongoing illness program. Until now, health insurance carriers have not encouraged Americans to remain healthy.

Abrogation of the Medical Rights of Bert Arenson

Returning to Bert Arenson of Cleveland, Ohio, his experience and current health difficulty are typical of the abrogation of a patient's rights. Because of years of effective suppression by the conspiracy of vested interests, Arenson was unaware of the existence of this treatment at the time chelation would have done him the most good — when he first began to get cardiac symptoms, in 1970. In this manner, his right to select and receive the treatment was substantially denied at that time.

Although he asked his cardiologist prior to bypass surgery whether he could find instead a metabolic treatment for what is, after all, a metabolic disease, the doctor did not inform him of the existence of any alternative and certainly said nothing about chelation therapy. It may have been a knowing refusal or simply ignorance on the part of his doctor. Again, Arenson's medical rights were effectively denied; in truth, he was *not* told what all of his choices were. And he is bitter about that.

When the patient did learn of the existence of chelation therapy, after the failure of bypass surgery, he had to travel 3,000 miles roundtrip for each of his first three courses of chelation treatment. This obviously entailed great expense and effort as well as risk in his unhealthy condition. Arenson obtained the treatment belatedly, but with extraordinary and unnecessary effort and expense. He told me, "During the two and a half years when I had to go out of town for the treatment, my wife and I spent a total of seven months in hotels."

Why Not Try Chelation Therapy Before Surgery?

An extremely important part of the conspiratorial suppression of chelation therapy is the refusal of Medicare, Blue Shield, and other third-party payers to compensate or reimburse for the treatment. The economic interests of medical orthodoxy are, of course, the most basic underpinning of this refusal. If chelation therapy was paid for by third party insurance, who would undertake vascular surgery without first trying chelation? Many of the heart surgeons and peripheral vascular surgeons would probably have to change their specialties.

More unfortunate than any other factor in this whole conspiracy, however, is that our own government is aiding the advancement of those medical financial interests above the interests of ordinary citizens. The financial drain on the average person can become quite serious. For patients without financial resources, it could mean denial of treatment and death.

How crazy the system is! Medicare is willing to pay ten to twenty-five times as much for bypass surgery as chelation therapy might cost. Nevertheless, the patient is directed toward surgery and away from chelation.

If chelation therapy hadn't faced this longtime, effective, and ruthless conspiracy, there would be more data, more experience, perhaps several double-blind studies, and a much greater background of research on the subject. There would be more facilities, more chelating physicians, and undoubtedly much lower costs. This would make the treatment more effective because it could be better tailored to the needs of you or me as the individual patient, with the development of more data. Our individual needs vary, but what never varies is our right to select the means by which we may preserve our bodies. That is our medical right — yours and mine! Should we be denied our medical right to take chelation therapy if we want it?

Chapter Fifteen

Our Medical Right to Chelation Therapy

Decisions about accepting/rejecting, withholding/withdrawing treatment are decisions (to be distinguished from diagnosis and prognosis) that whenever possible belong to the patient or, when the patient is incompetent, to those who presumably have the best interests of the patient at heart — saving right of appeal. This can easily be forgotten in a highly technological health-care system.

> Statement by Andre E. Hellegers, M.D., LeRoy Walters, James Childress, Rabbi Seymour Siegel, Richard A. McCormick, S.J., Roy Branson, Thomas Beauchamp, Seymour Perlin, M.D., and Joseph A. LaBarge (all members of the Kennedy Institute for the Study of Human Reproduction and Bioethics at Georgetown University), *The New York Times*, May 18, 1977

The Near-Death of Ophelia Clementino

For thirty years Palma C. Seders and her husband Amos have lived either with or close by Palma's parents in Temple City, California. The daughter watched gratefully as her mom and dad grew older gracefully together. Although they had their little illnesses, the old folks had many more ups than downs — until, that is, a few days after the seventy-ninth birthday of Palma's mother, Ophelia Clementino.

"My first indication of her illness," said Palma, "was during the first week of February, 1973. Momma came into the laundry room. On this particular morning I noted that she was incapable of operating the clothes washer. She seemed confused. The laundry was not properly sorted, and I had to help her with the task."

Palma observed her mother during the next few days and became alarmed at her incoherence and the obvious hallucinations she was experiencing. Then Palma made an appointment with Mrs. Clementino's personal physician in Pasadena, California. The doctor told them the problem was simply "old age."

This seemed an unsatisfactory diagnosis to the daughter, but she gave her mother the prescribed medication anyway. Severe and frequent headaches soon affected the patient.

Mrs. Clementino awoke at midnight on February 21, 1973 with one of those severe headaches. She looked pale, was upset, spoke incoherently, and acted unstable. Her doctor again examined her in the afternoon and decided that Mrs. Clementino had suffered a serious cerebrovascular accident (stroke). He recommended calling in a general practitioner who was located conveniently closer to the family's home. The second doctor confirmed the diagnosis and admitted the patient to the San Gabriel Valley Hospital.

Laboratory tests showed a blood clot had developed on the right side of the woman's head. It was causing some brain damage. Mrs. Clementino remained in the hospital and received treatment until allowed to return to Palma's home ten days later. There she was nursed by her daughter and a few other members of their large and loving family.

"Between May and September Momma suffered three more major strokes and several minor ones," Mrs. Seders related. "Each one left her more unstable and incoherent. By mid-October she had undergone a drastic change that was heartbreaking to see. She was no longer able to walk alone or write her name. Even her eating habits became abnormal. She ate with her fingers because she could not distinguish the silverware or was unable to hold it.

"It was twenty-four hours around the clock for dad and me watching my mother. She had to be pushed in the wheelchair because she couldn't comprehend how to operate it. She could not sleep without medication and remained awake much of the time. Her mind was fuzzy, which prevented her from realizing she couldn't stand alone, so she fell down at night when she attempted to go to the bathroom by herself.

"The afternoon that we had an appointment to see her new doctor," Mrs. Sedars continued, "my mother was struck again with a severe headache. I saw her color change, lips turned blue, and she trembled. The doctor said she was having another stroke. He injected Talwin (a pain killer) and sent me home with her to put her to bed. She remained there for two days except for the time she fell again and cut open her hand while attempting to go to the bathroom. A surgeon was called to stitch it.

"Then she had still another stroke. I recognized the signs, since her body turned limp and her skin became sallow, cold and clammy. She had no eyeball movement under the lids. She drifted into what appeared to be a coma. The doctor arrived many hours later and said Momma must be hospitalized as she had already begun to retain a lot of fluid and would soon develop pneumonia."

Mrs. Clementino was hospitalized for a second time in the San Gabriel Valley Hospital on November 12, 1973, where she was nursed by two of her daughters and other family members around the clock.

Ten days later the patient went home, but there she experienced another very serious stroke. This one contorted the right side of her face. It prevented her from swallowing even water without choking. The patient was paralyzed along her entire right side, including the throat muscles. Mrs. Seders tried to reach the doctor again by telephone.

"I explained to him what had happened and asked what more I could do for mother," she said. "He explained there was nothing he could tell me to do. He suggested that we should keep on making her as comfortable as possible and she would slowly slip away.

"As I replaced the receiver I sat there and wondered how long must this poor tortured soul go on like this — dying such a slow death? I would rather see my mother dead when I went back to her room than to have her suffer this way."

Dr. Harper Meets Mrs. Clementino

But Ophelia Clementino hung on to life for another three weeks. The whole family — her sons, daughters, daughters-in-law, sons-in-law, and husband — took turns nursing her. They gave her physical therapy three times a day. They fed her carefully by letting fluid trickle down the left side of her throat. Her throat muscles were too paralyzed for the use of a straw. They changed her diapers regularly, since she was incontinent and had lost control of her bowel sphincters. The matriarch was mindless — had no idea of where or who she was — and at times she thought Palma was her own mother.

Mrs. Clementino lost weight until she looked like the picture of death. She continued to suffer small strokes. For those who loved her, it was a heartbreaking time — a nightmare, they said. And even as the children worked to keep their mother alive, they agreed it would be better for Momma if she were already dead.

Al Clementino, Palma's younger brother, arrived with news about a doctor in Alabama who was having success treating patients for this same condition. Al telephoned H. Ray Evers, M.D. in Andalusia at the Columbia General Hospital. Dr. Evers listened to Al's description of his mother and determined that she was not strong enough for a flight to Alabama. He referred the family to Harold W. Harper, M.D., Director of the Harper Metabology and Nutrition Group in Los Angeles, California.

Dr. Harper returned the family's frantic call and consented to travel the thirty-eight miles from his office to Mrs. Seder's home, where the patient was being cared for. Dr. Harper asked that her medical and hospital records be acquired so that he could read them when he examined her. Four days later Palma had all of her mother's medical records. The physician arrived to examine his new patient on December 14, 1973.

"I'll always remember Mrs. Clementino," Dr. Harper told me. "Her ankles were swollen and fluid was in the base of her lungs. She was paralyzed on the right side; there was an absence of neurological responses on the right side — an absence of pulses also. Babinski reflex was negative; deep tendon reflexes were absent and she could not swallow; she could not hear. She could not speak or understand words either in English or Italian. The patient had no control of bowel movements; was semi-comatosed — lapsing in and out of sleep. The condition of her skin indicated a dehydrated condition. There was arrhythmia of the heart, overflowing medical evidence in all the parameters of the presence of arteriosclerotic disease; congestive heart failure with a free flux (swelling) of the lower extremities. My judgment was that Mrs. Clementino literally could have dropped dead at any moment."

Dr. Harper asked all the adult Clementino family members to gather together in the living room. "As we sat down I was sure he was thinking the same as were all of us — that it was almost too late for my mother," Palma Seders said. "Then for almost an hour he explained to us about chelation therapy — its meaning and purpose and the risks involved, since Momma was so far gone. We knew that the American medical profession did not approve of the procedure. Dr. Harper told us that. This meant that Medicare would not accept the financial burden. The treatment would probably be at our expense, without reimbursement from insurance. Therefore, it would incur much medical cost on our part. Momma would have to be hospitalized so there would be the risk of transporting her to the hospital by ambulance. There was the risk of losing her with the first treatment. She was so critical!"

"Yes, we discussed the dire emergency of the patient's condition," Dr. Harper later told me. "There was very little hope for her survival, no matter what modality she was treated with. One of the family members asked, 'Is there anything whatsoever that can be used to treat Momma?' In my medical opinion there was no therapy that would possibly give the patient even a chance, other than chelation therapy. Even with chelation, as I told the family that night, the patient might die before we could get her into the hospital. She might die after receiving the first chelation bottle, or the second. She might die in the middle of getting the treatment, or even at the end of it — because of her dire physical condition."

Silence lay heavy in that room. Seconds ticked by. The patient's children sat thinking. Then one of them said, "Neither one of her other doctors had any recommendations. They sent her home to die, and we can't accept that. Will you try to help her?"

Dr. Harper repeated his warnings about the closeness of death. He told them to think it over some more and if they wished to have their mother treated, yes, he would try to help.

That was a Friday night. The family telephoned the physician the following Sunday with the news that Momma Clementino had suffered her ninth stroke on Saturday morning. They thought surely she would die then, but this tenacious old lady still held onto life. What a will to live she possessed! She lingered through Sunday morning, and her children and husband decided they had to give her at least a fighting chance. The family begged the doctor to give her chelation treatment on Monday — if she survived until then.

The patient was transferred by ambulance from the Seders' home to St. Joseph's Hospital in Burbank, California, where Dr. Harper had provisional staff privileges. He was supervised by a medical staff advisor. In the hospital the physician's careful re-examination of Mrs. Clementino took much of Monday morning. She had been comatose now for several days. He ordered a full laboratory workup and medications for her. She also received oxygen.

In the afternoon Dr. Harper returned to read the patient's X-ray studies and to evaluate some of her laboratory test results. He did more of the same Tuesday and prescribed digitalis and diuretics to relieve her congestive heart failure and pulmonary edema. All of the various laboratory tests were completed by Friday morning.

Since the patient had remained in a stable condition, Dr. Harper ordered the first chelation treatment be given. He left complete written and oral instructions with the nurses on duty. The nursing staff members knew exactly how the solution was to be mixed — how much and the drops per minute. Dr. Harper had given unmistakable orders of what was to be done and how.

Mrs. Clementino Is Refused Chelation Therapy

Dr. Harper told the Clementino family that the first bottle of EDTA was going to be infused that day. "I wanted somebody from the family in attendance twenty-four hours a day," Dr. Harper said. "The lady needed full attention and the hospital couldn't spare around-the-clock nurses. The Clementinos were a very close-knit and loving family. They were anxious to help. Two of her children agreed to stay with the patient all the time."

Dr. Harper went back to see his patient and to make rounds Friday afternoon. Then he returned again after office hours Friday evening.

"I asked the two family members present what time the hospital staff had finished giving their mother the treatment," Dr. Harper explained. "And they said, 'Well they didn't bring anything in at all, doctor!' I was shocked! I said, 'What? Do you mean they didn't start the I.V. yet?'

" 'There's no I.V., doctor. They haven't given her anything!'

"Well, I flew out of that hospital room like a shot," said Dr. Harper, "and went to the nursing staion and shouted, 'why weren't my orders followed?' One of the nurses said, 'To find out, you'll have to see the nursing director!'

"I hunted her down," said the physician. "The nursing director told me she had been instructed not to follow my orders by the head of the experimental medicine committee of the hospital, who is a cardiologist. She told me I had to talk with him."

The Chairman of Experimental Medicine told Dr. Harper, "St. Joseph's Hospital really doesn't care what you give to your patients, doctor. If you want to take a tablet of arsenic and personally put it into the patient's mouth and wash it down with a glass of water because that's your way of practicing medicine, well — OK — you may poison anyone you wish as long as you take the entire responsibility. However, the nursing staff of St. Joseph's Hospital will not administer any of your poisons or other medications, because that implies that we approve of what you're doing, and we don't.

"You're new here, Dr. Harper — on provisional staff," continued the committee chief. "If you wish to give chelation therapy, you will have to sit there as every drop goes in; otherwise, it cannot be given in this hospital. We don't believe in that therapy or what you are doing with it."

Dr. Harper pointed out that it would take six hours or more for this particular patient to receive intravenous EDTA chelation for just one treatment. "I'll be happy to mix the solution and start the I.V. if I can save someone's life," he said, "but the family cannot afford to have me sit there for the whole time."

The hospital's experimental medicine committee chief remained unrelenting and refused any compromise. Dr. Harper was left dangling with his problem.

Palma Seders said, "The next thing for consideration was finding a place where this therapy could be administered. Dr. Harper was able to find a convalescent hospital where they agreed to permit chelation therapy. It was the best he could do. On December 22, 1973 Mom was discharged from St. Joseph's Hospital and transferred by ambulance to the Victory Convalescent Home in North Hollywood, California."

Palma Seders next described how she and the family members approached the situation. She told me in a long letter that the place was old and awful. The first thing the daughters did was to strip the bed, wash it with disinfectant, and order fresh linen. They cleaned the room and disinfected the furniture, too. The daughters agreed they were glad their mother was so incoherent and confused that she did not see the surroundings or understand what was taking place. Nevertheless, this was the only health facility available where anyone from the medical establishment would allow chelation therapy to be administered to the patient.

Unknown to the parties at that time, there was a single legal consequence of the patient's confinement in the convalescent home that would deprive Ophelia Clementino of Medicare reimbursement of her medical expenses. The reason was that she was not a patient in a certified hospital when Dr. Harper finally was able to administer EDTA to her.

The Patient Finally Receives Intravenous Chelation

"That North Hollywood convalescent home did not have a staff able to start the I.V.s, so I went there and mixed the solution and started the drip,"

Dr. Harper said. "The family members watched it go in and then told the nurses when it had finished. The nurses would enter the room and remove the I. V. needle and tubing. My plan was for a series of twenty-one chelation treatments administered every other day."

Palma Seders discussed the changes that started to take place. "It was after the third treatment that Momma started to recognize my sister Mary, Dad, and me," she told me. "She could swallow, too — not just liquids but solids."

"By the fifth treatment day," Dr. Harper related, "her neurological responses had begun to return to the right side. The Babinski reflex now became normal. By the six treatment day movement was noticed on the right side."

"He asked her to squeeze his hand," Palma said. "At first Momma refused for fear of hurting him. I told her to show Dr. Harper how strong she was by squeezing his hand. She did, and there was enough force in that weak little grip for the doctor to know she was responding. I could tell how pleased he was by the expression on his face. Mary, Dad and I were in tears. It was the first sign she had reflexes since November twenty-sixth. Now we felt some hope. To think that after all she had been through, perhaps now there would be a chance!"

Dr. Harper told me, "She began active movement of the right side of the body and was swallowing well by the eighth treatment day. She began to hold onto the bedside rail with her right hand and actively use it. I could communicate with her at that point very well."

Palma Seders added, "During the next four weeks Momma continued to make progress. Her improvement was remarkable. I took about 200 pictures of her during this time. By January fourth she looked great. The paralysis was completely gone. By January eleventh (the tenth chelation) she was able to use bedside facilities, brush her teeth, and eat by herself. It was amazing to watch how she took a cup of coffee and brought it to her mouth with her right hand. On January fourteenth, with our assistance she maneuvered herself to sit at the edge of the bed. Then we got her up in the wheelchair twice a day. Momma was doing so well that Dr. Harper felt we should try to get her on her feet, even if only to stand, to prepare her to relearn to walk. This she did with the aid of a walking device. She was quite proud of herself."

On the twelfth treatment day, the physician removed the indwelling catheter from Mrs. Clementino's bladder. She was continent and able to control her urinary flow. Her bowel movements had been controlled by the tenth treatment. By the sixteenth treatment the patient walked 150 yards by herself while using the walker. She doubled the distance by the eighteenth treatment, and finally she walked out of the home after the twenty-first treatment.

Two weeks after her discharge from the convalescent home, which had occurred February 6, 1974, Ophelia Clementino prepared to keep an appointment to see her physician. She anticipated it with excitement. A new hairdo was in order, she insisted, even for an eighty-two-year-old lady. Ophelia refused use of the walker because she wanted to walk into the doctor's office unaided on her own two feet. Her husband, her daughter Palma, and Palma's husband Amos, held their emotions in check as the elderly woman made her way through Dr. Harper's reception room door.

Palma told of the events of that day: "Now came what was to be one of the greatest days of my Mom's life, February eighteenth. She had a very restful night; she looked wonderful this morning; quite excited about getting to Dr. Harper's office. He hadn't seen her since she was discharged two weeks ago, and she had improved considerably.

"After breakfast I got her ready early so as to give us enough time to travel. We were to be at his office at 1:00 p.m. My husband stayed home from work that day to help me. He placed her wheelchair in the car and gave her the walker to help her outside. To my surprise she insisted she didn't need it anymore. She wanted to walk alone! We helped her into the car. I think we all tried to hold back our emotions. She looked just beautiful, and I took some snapshots of her as I always wanted to remember this moment.

"We arrived at the office at 12:30 p.m. I signed Mom in and told the doctor's receptionist that we were here. As we waited, Dr. Amy (Dr. Harper's associate) came out to the business office and noticed us seated in the waiting room. She had been at the convalescent hospital several times to give Mom some of her treatments. She rushed out into the waiting room to greet us and kissed my mother gently. Immediately she left the waiting room to tell Dr. Harper that we were here.

"Suddenly we looked up and out comes Dr. Harper! This was one of his very rare occasions to come out into the reception room. He put his strong arms around my Mom and kissed her tenderly. We could not hide our emotions.

"By now, everyone in the office knew who we were, even the patients who were waiting to see the doctor.

"As he examined her it was very obvious that he was quite pleased to see how much Mom had progressed in the past two weeks. He was rather surprised to hear that she walked without the use of the walker. We were to see him again March eighteenth.

"It was 5:00 p.m. when we left the doctor's office. I knew she was getting hungry, since we had eaten an early lunch. I told her we would be home soon and I would get our dinner ready. She turned to me and said I must be crazy to want to prepare dinner on such a wonderful day. My Mom wouldn't take no for an answer, so we ended up going out to dinner at her favorite coffee shop. She ate very well. We arrived home two hours later, and I was more tired out than was my Mom."

Following her original twenty-one chelations, Mrs. Clementino took five more treatments six months later and five further treatments six months after that. Nine months then passed without treatment, and she began showing signs of the return of her paralysis. Consequently, Dr. Harper administered ten additional chelation treatments — her last to date. The chelation therapy has kept the patient well and functional so far.

Mrs. Clementino is now well and carrying on a productive life. She vacuums, washes dishes, cooks, gardens, and is generally active in other ways in her own home. Her hearing has returned and her appetite is so good the family says she eats anything put in front of her, including Italian wine and sausage!

Ophelia Clementino's family refused to abandon their mother and give up her right to live with dignity. They rejected the medical establishment's advice to let her simply slip quietly into death. The woman owned a body, mind and spirit, and Palma, Frank, Mary, Al, Amos, Vickie, Joe, Dad and other family members did everything in their power to restore all three.

Every human being has that right. As long as a certain medical method exists that can be clinically applied to make a sick person function more normally, he or she, you or I, deserves the opportunity to receive that particular method. Regardless of cost or risk or criticism from orthodox organized medicine, we must demand our medical rights. Even if treatment has to be rendered in a motel, the back room of a pool hall, or in a broken-down convalescent home, as in Mrs. Clementino's case, it is our legal, moral, and ethical right to use our bodies as we see fit. It is also our constitutional right.

Ignorance of Treatment Is Malpractice

Alfred Soffer, M.D., Executive Director of the American College of Chest Surgeons says, "Unbridled therapeutic accessibility is not a service to the physician or patient, and the medical profession does not consider that unnecessary restrictions have been placed on it when worthless compounds are prohibited from sale and distribution. . . ."[1]

This is where Dr. Soffer's interpretation of the scientific method disagrees with the holistic concept of whole-person medical management.

George W. Kell, J.D., an attorney who practices law in Modesto, California, represented Ophelia Clementino in her fight for a Fair Hearing pursuant to Part B of the Medicare Act, after the carrier, Occidental Life Insurance Company of California, turned down her request for reimbursement of her medical bills. In his post-hearing brief, Attorney Kell wrote, "Had EDTA chelation therapy not been administered to the claimant she could not have survived more than a few days or at the outside, two to four weeks. EDTA chelation therapy was responsible for her recovery."[2]

According to Dr. Soffer's line of thinking, Mrs. Clementino should have been allowed to die. This attitude was also reflected by the second doctor Palma Seders called, who recommended that she should make her mother "as comfortable as possible and she would slowly slip away." Also, Dr. Soffer's kind of thinking is represented by the administration at St. Joseph's Hospital, which refused to permit hospital personnel to administer life-saving treatment. The various parties who represented the medical establishment condemned the patient to death, simply because they did not have knowledge of the treatment or did not like the therapy proposed.

In fact, both of Mrs. Clementino's former physicians, and St. Joseph's Hospital as well, had professional liability in her case. A court decision in California holds that every physician or hospital facility must explain *all* therapeutic alternatives. The California Supreme Court handed down that decision in the case of *Cobbs vs. Grant* (8 Cal 3d 229, 240; 104 C.R. 505, 513). The court said that every doctor owed the "duty of reasonable disclosure of the available choices with respect to proposed therapy and of the dangers inherently and potentially involved in each" to his patient.

The doctor or hospital that fails to deliver the best product for the patient, or withholds a therapy offering less danger to the patient, which the doctor or hospital has power to provide, may be held guilty of medical malpractice.

Cobbs vs. Grant further holds that a person of adult years and in sound mind, or his responsible agent, has the right, in the exercise of control over his own body, to determine upon his own course of treatment.

Ignorance of the treatment is also tantamount to malpractice, the court ruled. If the doctor or hospital *knew* of the alternative treatment and did not tell the patient, or her family, they, under the *Cobbs vs. Grant* informed-consent doctrine, would have every reason to sue. If the doctor or hospital did *not* know about chelation therapy, their ignorance of the method won't protect them if it is shown that, because of their ignorance, the patient has been deprived of treatment alternatives.

The Physician's Right to Practice Nontoxic Medicine

"Nontoxic drugs can be deadly because their use may cause delay in instituting correct therapy," Dr. Soffer also said.[1] But no other life-saving therapy had been instituted or even suggested for the dying patient. The administration of EDTA therapy was absolutely necessary and reasonable, Attorney Kell argued. Mrs. Clementino would not be alive otherwise. It is the role of the physician to extend life if possible, and to make what remains of life more comfortable if possible. The reason this patient did not die is because of chelation therapy alone, the attorney said, and for no other reason.

Mr. Kell also argued that under the case of *People vs. Montecino* (66 Cal App 2d 85; 152 P 2d 5; 10 ALR 1137), a doctor is potentially subject to criminal liability if he fails to administer a curative substance, resulting in the dealth or injury of the patient. As to his patient, Ophelia Clementino, Dr. Harper testified, "This woman would have undoubtedly died if the therapy had been withheld."

As was noted above, under *Cobbs vs. Grant*, a doctor is required under penalty of being found guilty of malpractice to inform his patient of all available modalities of treatment. The patient then has the right to make an informed decision as to which therapy the patient will elect to receive. Dr. Harper acted honorably and so informed the Clementino family, the patient's representatives. The family made its decision, and the physician then had no alternative except to comply with the family members' choice of treatment. Had he failed to provide chelation therapy, or had he failed to advise the family of its availability, the doctor would have been guilty of malpractice under that rule of law. Had Dr. Harper failed to provide the therapy, it would have meant the abandonment of the woman.

Thus Mr. Kell advised, "A physician who is following his conscience must use whatever modality is necessary in order to sustain the life of the patient in as comfortable and as functional a way as possible. This would include chelation therapy or anything else, regardless of whether the therapy is generally recognized or not."

Attorney Kell told the Fair Hearing Officer, Attorney Curtis L. Klahs of Glendale, California, that with respect to the use of drugs authorized for *one* purpose, and under some conditions used for *another* purpose, "there is no medical prohibition against such use by a practicing and qualified physician."

The drug's package insert only sets up guidelines for the use of the medication, not parameters, he argued. Attorney Kell cited Valium as an example. "Valium is licensed as a tranquilizer, but is often prescribed as a sedative," he said. "Several hundred drugs are commonly used in this way in American medical practice, although the use is not specifically listed on the drug enclosure."[2] That was the common practice in Dr. Harper's community, as it is in the communities of most physicians around the country. Additionally, this practice has the sanction of the FDA itself. The FDA has sent letters to that effect to H. Ray Evers, M.D.

One more thing regarding the physician's right to practice medicine according to his conscience: the doctor has the right and duty to treat any patient who is suffering from morbidity, lack of appetite, weight loss, pain, the potential of imminent death, or other malfunctions. He must use his best judgment in doing so to accomplish the purpose for which he is employed. How does the doctor justify himself or protect himself from incrimination by medical colleagues, health insurance carriers, governmental agencies, and other involved parties when — even though he has been able to bring about the alleviation or cure of various conditions — he is attacked by his colleagues because he has treated with a medication that is frowned upon or disapproved? Must he face going to jail, or be threatened with forfeiture of his license, as happened to H. Ray Evers, M.D. of Montgomery, Alabama in the first instance, or Robert J. Rogers, M.D. of Melbourne, Florida in the second?

The Federal Ruling Against Mrs. Clementino

Elderly Mrs. Clementino did not succeed in her pursuit of a "Fair Hearing." Attorney George Kell pointed to the evidence that overwhelmingly established the reasonableness and necessity of chelation therapy in her case at her "Fair Hearing." That was all that the Medicare recipient was allowed under Part B.

Mr. Kell said, "Ophelia Clementino would have been dead within hours or days at the most, and as additional treatments were administered she continued to prosper in her health, from day to day and from week to week. Thus, to hold that she should have been denied the benefit of this treatment because it does not, in the opinion of some experts, constitute a 'specific or effective treatment for the particular condition' from which she was suffering, would amount to a denial of her right to life."[3]

Mr. Kell argued into a vacuum, for Hearing Officer Klahs denied the beneficiary's claim under Part B of Medicare. And she could not collect under Part A because her treatment was given in a convalescent home and not in a regular hospital. Remember, she had to be moved out of St. Joseph's Hospital in order for the patient to receive the treatment of her doctor's choice.

Attorney Klahs wrote: "It has been found by this Hearing Office that chelation therapy with endate [sic] disodium (EDTA) is not *reasonable and necessary* in treating the beneficiary's diagnosed condition. Therefore, this treatment is not covered under the Medicare program and was properly disallowed by the Carrier [emphasis added].

"It has further been found by this Hearing Officer that the diagnostic procedures relating to the chelation therapy treatment were not *reasonable and necessary* and therefore were not covered under the Medicare program and properly disallowed by the Carrier."[4]

Strangely enough, the Medicare Act, Part B provides that there shall be no appeal from this "Fair Hearing" decision, although under Part A of the Act an appeal is allowed for the identical services. In a Part A appeal from a Hearing Officer's prior decision denying payment for a chelation hospital confinement, D. D. Dominey won his appeal. Attorney Kell cited the Dominey case in his brief. He argued that it should be followed in Mrs. Clementino's Part B case because the facts were identical. If Mr. Dominey was entitled to relief under Part A so was Mrs. Clementino entitled to relief under Part B of the Medicare Act. But the argument was ignored by Mr. Klahs. The technicality of the Victory Convalescent Hospital not being a regular hospital may have been a factor here, but Mr. Klahs did not state that one way or another. He just ignored the Dominey precedent.

This adverse ruling for the Medicare Part B recipient occurred despite the enactment of guidelines under Section 2050.1 of the *Hearing Officer's Coverage and Limitations Handbook*. These guidelines have no standing as a statute and tell only of procedure to be followed. These guidelines can be changed to fit the case, but Mr. Klahs offered a deaf ear, a blind eye and a closed mind. Section 2050.1 states:

Endrate (*Chelating Agent*) — Based on the Food and Drug Administration's evaluation, the intravenous injection of disodium edetate is indicated in selected patients for the emergency treatment of *hypercalcemia* and *for the control of ventricular arrhythmias and heart block associated with digitalis toxicity*.

A guideline is, by definition, no more than a guideline. Mr. Kell quoted from Webster's Dictionary as follows:

A line by which one is guided, as: (a) a cord or rope to aid a passer over a difficult point or to permit retracing a course; (b) an *indication* or *outline* (as by a government) of policy or conduct. [emphasis added]

Interpreting that definition, the attorney's brief suggested that the guideline provided an "indication," but is not conclusively determinative of an issue. Thus, Mr. Kell argued, Klahs should have ruled according to the circumstances, under which the beneficiary had been barely surviving *before* she received chelation therapy and the undisputed fact that this treatment had saved her life. But no, Hearing Officer Klahs did not see fit to vary from the strict letter of the medical establishment's guideline.[3]
Another portion of Section 2050.1 states:

Injections Not Specifically Indicated. — Payment should not be made for injections which are not considered by accepted standards of medical practice to be indicated as a specific or effective treatment for the particular condition for which they are given (although the injection may be accepted treatment for another illness). . . .

The key word in this guideline, obviously, is *should*. If the guideline were intended to have the force and effect of law it would necessarily provide that "payment *shall* not be made . . ." Thus we see that, by its own terms, the guideline itself is not conclusive as to its application, but is only meant to provide a serviceable guide for use in the absence of substantial evidence to the contrary. Mr. Kell's brief argued that this guideline conforms to Congressional intent by permitting the hearing officer to award payment in those cases wherein injections are in fact shown to be "reasonable or necessary for the diagnosis or treatment of illness or injury," as provided by Section 1862 (a) of the Medicare Act (Title XVIII of the Social Security Act). But the point was simply ignored by Klahs' decision, which ritualistically cited the "hypercalcemia/ventricular arrhythmias and heart block" formula as its basis for denial.

Non-Payment for Chelation by Medicare Denies Due Process
Ophelia Clementino is an example of but one more U.S. citizen and beneficiary of the Medicare Act who was denied the right of due process.

The medical rights of chelated patients have been abrogated illegally. The Federal officials or private carriers who decided against payment of bills for chelation therapy are taking upon themselves the control over what kind of medicine the patient should receive.

Under Section 1801 of the Medicare Act it is provided that:

> Nothing in this Title shall be construed to authorize any Federal officer or employee to exercise any supervision or control over the practice of medicine or the manner in which medical services are provided . . ."

Where Section 2050.1 of the Hearing Officer's Guidelines attempts to declare ineffective that which is *shown* to have been effective, as in the particular patients whom I have described, the guideline amounts to nothing less than a covert attempt on the part of Federal agents to exercise the forbidden supervision or control over the practice of medicine, and the method of practice of that profession. For these reasons the guideline, where it is preferred by a hearing officer over the provisions of the Act requiring payment for reasonable and necessary services, constitutes a denial of the right of due process for all these patients. What possible compelling governmental interest exists, for example, to justify the denial of EDTA therapy in the case of Ophelia Clementino?

As indicated, the Hearing Officer's guidelines say: ". . . disodium edetate is indicated in selected patients for the emergency treatment of hypercalcemia and . . . ventricular arrhythmias and heart block associated with digitalis toxicity."

In his testimony about Mrs. Clementino's condition, Dr. Harper said that arteriosclerosis is caused by deposits of mineral and arterial plaques in the arteries and veins of the patient. Chelation therapy was given to her in order to cause a chelate to form between the mineral deposit on the arterial wall and the chelating agent itself, and thus improve her vascular circulation. The calcium deposits in this lady's arteries and veins, and throughout the cells of her body, were abnormal. Such an abnormality is a hypercalcemic condition. It was this abnormality which resulted in her arteriosclerotic disease.

"As a physician, I am not able to prevent the EDTA from affecting the arteriosclerosis in the process of chelating for excess minerals, such as calcium," said Dr. Harper. "Hypercalcemia is a *laboratory finding*, rather than a disease."

"The removal of excess calcium deposits by the EDTA chelation therapy," said Attorney Kell, "was the specific which preserved this patient's life. There could not be anything more specific or effective." (There is one other effective chelating drug marketed in the Orient, but it is not available in the West. It is called *anginen*, an oral tablet produced by the Japanese.)

Therefore, the argument that chelation therapy is not compensable because of the provision of the guidelines which allow only for its use in cases of "hypercalcemia" and digitalis intoxication is shown to be in error. (*Digital-*

is intoxication is a poisoning of the patient caused by too large a dose.) Furthermore, since its use for hypercalcemia is allowed, and since arteriosclerosis consists of excessive plaques containing calcium, other minerals, waste products, and fat deposits, then it must be clear that the use of EDTA infusion for the removal of the calcium deposits constitutes a proper treatment.

Why is chelation therapy authorized for the treatment of a laboratory finding, *hypercalcemia*, and not for the related disease process, *atherosclerosis*? Proper interpretation of the guidelines would be that chelation therapy is authorized for the removal of excessive calcium deposits where these, alone or in conjunction with other material, threaten the health and well-being of a patient. Atherosclerosis happens to be an associated finding and, in fact, is an integral part of the disease. Thus we see that, even under the existing guidelines, the treatment with EDTA chelation must be authorized. Those patients denied this authorization are having their medical rights nullified. This is a violation of human rights that is now occurring regularly in this country, I am sorry to report.

Medical Rights Groups Form

Realizing that vested interests are attempting to take away the right of the patient to receive, or for a physician to administer, chelation therapy, a number of medical rights groups are forming. For example, Hugo Loseke of Sebastian, Florida doesn't think the government has any business telling him whether he can or cannot take the therapy. Loseke, age fifty-eight, owns a construction firm. He has organized the National Association for Freedom of Medical Choice. Along with fifty other members of this Brevard County group, Loseke believes he has a constitutional right to receive any medical treatment he or his fellow members and their physicians agree upon.

"We're scared to death we won't be able to get chelation," said Loseke, who has arteriosclerosis. "It just boils down to one fact. If my physician and I decide on a treatment, nobody else should have a say in it."

In Hartford, Connecticut in the fall of 1978, the Association for Cardiovascular Therapies, Inc. was formed with Audrey Goldman as secretary-treasurer, Alvin Kavaler as vice president, and myself as president. Our intent is to perform a public service by furnishing information on chelating physicians in local areas. The office is located at 1845 Summer Street, Stamford, Connecticut 06905.

Since current medical practice does not subscribe to the chelation therapeutic technique, we created the Association for Cardiovascular Therapies (A.C.T.) to encourage this and other more holistic approaches. A.C.T. suggests that medical attention should be rendered to the whole person and take into account his body, mind, spirit, and emotions. It endorses the finding of an improved delivery system for the preservation of human life and health. It encourages two facets of improvement: first, the individual must take responsibility for personal health; and second, every available therapy, including alternatives to traditional treatments, should be tried. Chelation therapy is among those alternatives.

A.C.T. endeavors to protect the physician/patient relationship against government or other outside intervention. It also attempts to increase reimbursement and expand coverage by third-party health insurance for alternative therapies. A.C.T. members pay $15 annual dues and work to educate legislators and other government officials about the many techniques useful to alter cardiovascular degeneration — reverse hardening of the arteries — among the populace. We conduct seminars and publish a quarterly newsletter describing advances in cardiovascular care, preventive medicine, diagnosis, and treatment.

The Connecticut contingent of A.C.T. is patterned after the Association for Chelation Therapy, created seven years ago by Mrs. Collie Green of San Gabriel, California. The California Association for Chelation Therapy (ACT) is a tax-exempt corporation that disseminates information about chelation therapy.

ACT is helping to defend physicians against the legal, financial, and peer pressures of the medical establishment. The Association has successfully defended Donald E. Medaris, M.D. of Pasadena, California. Dr. Medaris practices internal medicine and specializes in cardiovascular diseases for which he uses chelation therapy. He had been harassed by the California State Board of Medical Examiners for his patient treatment with intravenous infusion of EDTA.

Mrs. Greene has close personal knowledge of chelation therapy's value and that is the reason she formed ACT. She wishes to help others avoid the harrowing events that she and her husband had undergone before turning to chelation therapy.

He Had No Alternative

At 6:30 a.m. on February 3, 1973, forty-eight-year-old Robert E. Greene of San Gabriel, California was rushed by firemen to his community's coronary care unit (CCU). Doctors there diagnosed his chest pain as acute myocardial infarction. He was treated and his life saved. After he returned home from three weeks of hospitalization, Dr. Greene's heart did not seem much better, though, and this caused him to worry. His overriding questions were, "Where do I go from here? Will there be any kind of life for me? How do I avoid having a heart attack again?"

For answers, the patient's cardiologist recommended the standard course for heart attack victims, a full cardiac study, including coronary arteriography. The evaluation and his arteriogram were carried out at the Rancho Los Amigos Hospital, the University of Southern California Medical Center in Downey, California.

Dr. Greene and his wife Collie listened to findings afterward which left them stunned. The patient had triple blood vessel involvement. Two of his coronary arteries were totally occluded and another artery was 80 percent occluded. Forty percent of the man's left heart ventricle had turned to scar tissue, due to the massive heart attack. Severe damage caused the blood that nourished the heart to have slowed to a trickle.[5]

"The panel of doctors who studied my husband explained that he could not live in this condition," said Collie Greene. "They said his only hope of survival was surgery. They would do a resectioning of the heart and a double bypass. They thought it would also be absolutely necessary to remove the damaged tissue from the heart muscle. Essentially, this was two different heart operations.

"We asked about the success of such an operation," the wife recalled. "But the doctors had no information to give on this type of surgery because it had only been done at their major hospital for three years. We did talk at length about the risks involved. They said there would be a thirty percent chance of death for my husband with such an operation. When asked about being able to return to his present position [as a corporate personnel director] the doctors were in doubt. They felt that the load my husband was carrying — recruiting, lecturing, and meetings that went with his full-time job — would be too much for him after such a delicate operation." Mrs. Greene added, "To us the recommendations seemed more like an omen of death rather than a hope of survival.

"We asked for alternatives. It being a research center, we thought the panel of Rancho Los Amigos doctors would have some answers for us. We were told that there were no alternatives. No alternatives? We were shaken! Then we started to beg — we pleaded — and we were told again, 'There are *no* alternatives!'

"It was the middle of May, and the panel suggested that if Bob were still alive we should return to Rancho Los Amigos Hospital again in September to discuss further the question of surgery. We felt such hopelessness, such despair and very much alone," she shuddered.

"As we left the room almost stumbling in a daze, a doctor walked out with us. He advised us to face reality. 'Go home, make your will, and put your house in order. No matter what you do, the situation is a dismal one,' he said. We went home and took this doctor's advice. We set out to put our affairs in order. It was an ordeal for the whole family to tend to these necessary tasks," Mrs. Greene remembered. "Then we decided to look for alternatives on our own. After two weeks of searching, we found out about chelation therapy."

The entire Greene family and many of their friends had put in what seemed like endless telephone calls to all parts of the United States. They were looking for *some* kind of alternative to open-heart surgery, where the risk of death for Robert Greene would not be so high. They found an alternative in the little-known intravenous EDTA chelation procedure. The patient took the therapy.

"In about four months my husband returned to work full time, to the same position. He is responsible for two thousand people. He is able to do all the traveling, lecturing, and everything necessary to fulfull his job. He has been able to take all the stress and strain that this type of work entails," said Mrs. Greene.

"He has made a total commitment to the full treatment regimen that goes with chelation, as his doctors repeatedly request it of patients. He had to change his lifestyle and especially his eating patterns. This has been stressed over and over again," she said.

"My husband walks nearly four miles an hour now. He rides his bicycle twelve miles in an hour. He enjoys all the sports, and he enjoys being able to go back to sailing." Mrs. Greene smiled, "Bob keeps telling us that sailing takes very little effort, and according to his pulse rate, it really does."

Robert Greene joined a cardiac rehabilitation program at Ranchos Los Amigos Hospital in December, 1973 and now routinely plays three games of vigorous volleyball. By April 1980, he had taken almost eighty chelation treatments in a regular maintenance program. He has enjoyed seven active, happy, and fulfilling years from the time his imminent death was forecast in 1973. His only legacy of that time is a massive scar in his heart — and some unhappy memories of orthodox medicine's stubborn refusal to sanction chelation therapy.

Collie Greene has founded and is the current director of the Association for Chelation Therapy, because the treatment is hardly known in the United States, even among physicians — to say nothing of the public. It is the only alternative to progressive arterial degeneration — the *one* proven means by which a person can prevent or quickly reverse hardening of the arteries. Her organization is formed to educate the public and the doctors that atherosclerosis can be reversed through chelation therapy.

Mrs. Greene added, "We are really pleased that we did not accept the surgery. We are very fortunate to have found chelation. We feel this therapy has, indeed, given my husband a new life."

In my last contact with Collie Green before I finalized this chapter, she said, "As I reflect on our experiences, I still shudder at the thought that we almost made the vital decision for Bob to have open heart surgery when we were in such total ignorance and fear. I keep asking myself, why did we have to live a nightmare that way? Why were we not informed of alternatives when we begged for them? The doctors said, 'There are no alternatives.' But they lied! If a physician does not know of treatment alternatives, why in the world doesn't he seek them out for the sake of his patient? If he does know about them, then he must tell you what else you can do before undergoing something so hazardous as open heart surgery or other surgery. Perhaps with publication of your book everyone in the country — in the world — will know that hardening of the arteries can be reversed by chelation therapy. Now there will be no excuse not to be informed."

Mrs. Greene concluded: "What keeps going through my mind is that the patient has the right to be informed of any alternatives, regardless of the personal opinion of the physician toward those alternatives. This is the right of the patient, and he must not be denied this right."

Now, It Is Up To You

This is the right of the patient, and he must not be denied this right. Those words by Collie Green summarize my own feelings regarding chelation therapy. I know that, today, virtually all of my friends and family — in fact, virtually every American adult — suffers from some hardening of the arteries. This disease will kill more than one million Americans this year; millions more will face restricted lifestyles, heavy medical bills, and even costly and dangerous surgery because of this epidemic disease.

And yet, as I have learned, hardening of the arteries *can be prevented or reversed*. A safe, simple, and inexpensive treatment called chelation therapy could perform medical miracles in this country, if only it were understood, accepted, and properly promoted. We would live longer, healthier, happier lives.

There are powerful forces at work in our country to suppress this important medical discovery. For many different reasons — united only by a combination of ignorance, arrogance, and greed — the medical establishment, the political establishment, drug companies, and the health insurance industry have combined to deny this treatment to you and your loved ones.

A few courageous physicians have defied the powers-that-be to promote chelation therapy. Thousands of desperate patients have proven to themselves the life-saving benefits of this treatment. It is up to us to make certain that more Americans learn of it. It is for this reason that I have written this book. Now, it is up to you.

Footnotes

Chapter One
[1] Clark, Matt and Greenberg, Peter S. "Riddled by isotopes." *Newsweek*, March 21, 1977.
[2] Wolinsky, Howard: "Area man: treatment restored vision." *Today*, January 9, 1977.
[3] Ibid.

Chapter Three
[1] Alsleben, H. Rudolph, and Shute, Wilfrid E.: *How to Survive the New Health Catastrophes*. Anaheim, California: Survival Publications, Inc., 1973.

Chapter Four
[1] Gordon, T.; Kannel, W. B.; and Sorlie, P. D. "The Framingham Study." National Institutes of Health, May 1971.
[2] Holling, N. E. *Peripheral Vascular Diseases*. Philadelphia: J. B. Lippincott Company, 1972.
[3] Keys, A. "Coronary heart disease in seven countries." *Circulation 41*: 1 (1970).
[4] Keys, A., et al. "Probability of middle-aged men developing coronary heart disease in five years." *Circulation 45* (1972), 815.
[5] Enos, W. F.; Beyer, J. C.; and Holmes, R. H. "Pathogenesis of coronary disease in American soldiers killed in Korea." *J.A.M.A. 158* (1955), 912-914.
[6] McNamara, J. J., et al. "Coronary artery disease in combat casualties in Vietnam." *J.A.M.A. 216* (1971), 1185-1187.
[7] Brucknerova, O., and Tulacek, J. "Chelates in the treatment of occlusive atherosclerosis." *Vnitr. Lek. 18* (1972), 729.
[8] Kurliandchikov, V. N. "Treatment of patients with coronary arteriosclerosis with Unithiol in combination with decamevit." *Vrach. Delo. 6* (1973), 8.
[9] Ohno, T. "Clinical and experimental studies of arteriosclerosis." *Exerpta Medica: Intern. Med. 17*: 8 (1963).
[10] Seven, M. J. (ed.). *Metal Binding in Medicine*. Philadelphia: J. B. Lippincott Company, 1960.
[11] Soffer, A. *Chelation Therapy*. Springfield, Illinois: Charles G. Thomas, Publisher, 1964.
[12] Spencer, H. "Studies on the effects of chelating agents in man." *Ann. N.Y. Acad. Sci. 88* (1960), 435.
[13] Clarke, N. E.; Clarke, C. N.; and Mosher, R. E. "Treatment of angina pectoris with disodium ethylene diamine tetraacetic acid." *Am. J. Med. Sc. 232* (1956), 654-666.
[14] Kitchell, J. R., et al. "The treatment of coronary artery disease with disodium EDTA — A reappraisal." *Am. J. Cardiol. 11* (1963), 501-506.
[15] Lamar, C. P. "Calcium chelation of atherosclerosis — nine years' clinical experience." Fourteenth Annual Meeting, American College of Angiology, 1968.

[16] Meltzer, L. E.; Urol, M. E.; and Kitchell, J. R. "The treatment of coronary artery disease with disodium EDTA." In Seven, M. J. (ed.) *Metal Binding in Medicine.* Philadelphia: J. B. Lippincott Company, 1960, pp. 132-136.

[17] Boyle, A. J., et al. "Studies in human and induced atherosclerosis." *J.Am. Geriatr. Soc. 14* (1966), 272.

[18] Lamar, C. P. "Chelation endarterectomy for occlusive atherosclerosis." *J. Am. Geriatr. Soc. 14* (1966) 272.

[19] Lamar, C. P. "Chelation therapy of occlusive arteriosclerosis in diabetic patients." *Angiology 15* (1965), 379.

[20] Nikitina, E. K., et al. "Treatment of atherosclerosis with trilon B. (EDTA)." *Kardiologiia 12* (1972), 137.

[21] Olwin, J. H., and Koppel, J. L. "Reduction of elevated plasma lipid levels in atherosclerosis following EDTA therapy." *Proc. Soc. Exp. Biol. Med. 128* (1968), 1137-1139.

[22] Klevay, L. M. "Coronary heart disease: zinc/copper hypothesis." *Am. J. Clin. Nutr. 28* (1975), 764-774.

[23] Zapadnick, V. I., et al. "Pharmacological activity of Unithiol and its use in clinical practice." *Vrach. Delo. 8* (1973), 122.

[24] Soffer, A. "Chelation therapy for arteriosclerosis." *J.A.M.A. 233* (1975).

[25] Craven, P. C., and Morelli, H. F. "Chelation therapy." *West. J. Med. 122* (1975), 277-278.

[26] "CMA warns against chelation." *CMA News 20:* 13, Sept. 12, 1975, p. 3.

[27] Pullman, T. N., et al. "Synthetic chelating agents in clinical medicine." In DeGraff, A. D. (ed.) *Annual Review of Medicine.* Calif.: Annuals Reviews, 1963.

[28] James, T. N. "Selective experimental chelation of calcium in the sinus mode." *J. Mol. Cell. Cardiol. 6* (1975), 493-504.

[29] Isaacs, J. P., and Lamb, J. C. "Trace metals, vitamins, and hormones in ten-year treatment of coronary atherosclerotic heart disease." Library of Congress Catalog Card Number 74-82883, as delivered at the Texas Heart Institute Symposium on Coronary Artery Medicine and Surgery, Houston, Texas. February 21, 1974.

[30] Soffer, A.; Toribara, T.; and Sayman, A. "Myocardial responses to chelation." *Br. Heart J. 23* (1961), 690-694.

[31] Soffer, A., et al. "Clinical applications and untoward reactions of chelation in cardiac arrhythmia." *Arch. Intern. Med. 106* (1960), 824-834.

[32] Popovic, A., et al. "Experimental control of serum calcium levels *in vivo.*" Georgetown University Medical Center. *Proc. Soc. Exp. Biol. Med. 74* (1950), 415-417.

[33] Rubin, M. "Fifth Conference on Metabolic Interrelations." *Biologic Action of Chelating Agents.* Macy Foundation, 1954, pp., 344-358.

[34] Hastings, A. B. "Studies on the effect of alteration of calcium in circulating fluids on the mobility of calcium." *Trans. Macy Conf. Metabolic Interrelations 3* (1951), 38-50.

[35] Friedman, H. "The significance of Mg/Ca ratio." Ph.D. thesis, Graduate Department of Chemistry, Georgetown University, 1952.

Chapter Five

[1] Gordon, Garry F., and Vance, Robert B. "EDTA chelation therapy for arteriosclerosis: history and mechanisms of action." *Osteopathic Annals 4:* 38-62, February 1976.

[2] Demesy, F., "On the mechanism of papaverine action on the control of vascular smooth muscle contractile activity by extracellular calcium." *J. Pharm. Pharmacol, 23* (1971), 712, 713.

[3] Triner, L., et al. "Cyclic phosphodiestasterase activity and the action of papaverine." *Biochem. Biophys. Res. Commun. 40* (1970). 64-69.

[4] Greengard, P., et al. *Advances in Cyclic Nucleotide Research*, Volume 1. New York: Raven Press, 1972, pp. 195-211.

[5] Sivjakov, K. I. "The treatment of acute selenium, cadmium and tungsten intoxication in rats with calcium disodium ethylene diamine tetraacetate." *Toxicol. Appl. Pharmacol. 1* (1959), 602-608.

[6] Tessinger, J. "Biochemical responses to provocative chelation by edatate disodium calcium." *Arch. Environ. Health 23* (1971), 280.

[7] Klevay, L. M. "Coronary heart disease: zinc/copper hypotheses." *Am. J. Clin. Nutr. 28* (1975), 764-774.

[8] Schroeder, H. A. *The Poisons Around Us*. Bloomington, Ind.: Indiana University Press, 1974.

[9] Freemen, R. "Reversible myocarditis due to chronic lead poisoning in childhood." *Arch. Dis. Child. 40* (1965), 389-393.

[10] Price, J. M. "Some effects of chelating agents on tryptophan metabolism in man." *Fed. Proc.* (Suppl. 10, 1961), 223-226.

[11] Petersdorf, R. G. "Internal medicine in family practice." *N. Engl. J. Med. 293* (1975), 326.

[12] Malmstron, B. G. "Role of metal binding in enzymic reactions." *Fed. Proc.* (Suppl. 10, 1961), 60-69.

[13] Zelis, R., et al. "Effects of hyperlipoproteinemias and their treatment on the peripheral circulation." *J. Clin. Invest. 49* (1970), 1007.

[14] Sincock, A. "Life extension in the rotifer by application of chelating agents." *J. Gerontol. 30* (1975), 289-293.

[15] Blankenhorn, D. H., and Bolwick, L. E. "A quantitive study of coronary arterial calcification." *Am. J. Pathol. 39* (1961), 511.

[16] Schroeder, H. A., and Perry, H. M., Jr. "Antihypertensive effects of binding agents." *J. Lab. Clin. Med. 46* (1955), 416.

[17] Shin, Yeh Yu. "Cross-linking of elastin in human atherosclerotic aertas." *Lab. Invest. 25* (1971), 121.

[18] Hall, D. A. "Coordinately bound calcium as a cross-linking agent in elastin and as an activator of elastolysis." *Gerontologia 16* (1970), 325-339.

[19] Wilder, D. A. "Mobilization of atherosclerotic plaque calcium with EDTA utilizing the isolation-persusion principle." *Surgery 52* (1962), 5.

[20] Schreiber, G. "*In vivo* thinning of thickened capillary basement membranes by rapid chelation." (unpublished manuscript).

[21] Boyle, A. J.; Mosher, R. E.; and McCann, D. S. "Some vivo effects of chelation. 1: Rheumatoid arthritis." *J. Chronic Dis. 16* (1963), 325-328.

[22] Leipzig, L. H.; Boyle, A. J.; and McCann, D. S. "Case histories of rheumatoid arthritis treated with sodium or magnesium EDTA." *J. Chronic Dis. 22* (1970), 553-563.

[23] Uhl, H. S. M., et al. "Effect of EDTA on cholesterol metabolism in rabbits." *Am. J. Clin. Pathol. 23* (1953), 1226-1233.

[24] Jacob, H. S. "Pathologic states of erythrocyte membrane." University of Minnesota. *Hospital Practice*, pp. 47-49, December, 1974.

[25] Soffer, A.; Toribara, T.; and Sayman, A. "Myocardial response to chelation." *Br. Heart J. 23* (1961), 690-694.

[26] Soffer, A., et al. "Clinical applications and untoward reactions of chelation in cardiac arrhythmias." *Arch. Intern. Med. 166* (1960), 824-834.

[27] Perry, H. M., Jr. "Hypertension and the geochemical environment." *Ann. N.Y. Acad. Sci. 199* (1972), 202-228.

[28] Popvic, A., et al. "Experimental control of serum calcium levels *in vivo*." Georgetown University Medical Center. *Proc. Soc. Exp. Biol. Med. 74* (1950), 415-417.

29 Lamar, C. P. "Calcium chelation of atherosclerosis — nine years; clinical experience." Fourteenth Annual Meeting, American College of Angiology, 1968.

30 Meltzer, L. E.; Urol, M. E.; and Kitchell, J. R. "The treatment of coronary artery disease with disodium EDTA." In Seven, M. J., (ed.) *Metal Binding in Medicine*. Philadelphia: J. B. Lippincott Co., 1960, pp. 132-136.

31 Meltzer, L. E., et al. "The urinary excretion pattern of trace metals in diabetes mellitus." *Am. J. Med. Sci.* 244 (1962), 282-289.

32 Kitchell, J. R.; Meltzer, L. E.; and Seven, M. J. "Potential uses of chelation methods in the treatment of cardiovascular diseases." *Prog. Cardiovasc. Dis.* 19 (1961), 798.

33 Bjorksten, J. "Crosslinking and the aging process." In Rockstein, M. (ed.). *Theoretical Aspects of Aging*. New York: Academic Press, 1974.

34 Koen, A.; McCann, D. S.; and Boyle, A. J. "Some *in vivo* effects of chelation. II: Animal experimentation." *J. Chronic Dis.* 16 (1963), 329-333.

35 Kitchell, J. R.; Meltzer, L. E.; and Rutman, E. "Effects of ions on *in vitro* gluconeogenesis in rat kidney cortex slices." *Am. J. Physiol.* 208 (1965), 841-846.

36 Strain, W. H., et al (eds.) *Clinical Application of Zinc Metabolism*. Springfield, Ill.: Charles C. Thomas, Publisher, 1974.

37 Friedman, M. *Pathogenesis of Coronary Artery Disease*. San Francisco: McGraw-Hill, 1969.

38 Zohman, B. "Emotional factors in coronary disease." *Geriatrics* 28 (1973), 110.

39 Miller, In Strain, W. H., et al. (eds.): *Clinical Application of Zinc Metabolism*. Springfield, Ill.: Charles C. Thomas, 1974.

40 Peters, H. A. "Trace minerals, chelating agents and the porphyrias." *Fed. Proc.* (Suppl. 10, 1961), 227-234.

41 Timmerman, A., and Kallistatos, G. "Modern aspects of chemical dissolution of human renal calculi by irrigation." *J. Urol.* 95 (1966), 469-475.

42 Birk, R. E., and Rupe, C. E. "The treatment of systemic sclerosis with EDTA, pyridoxine and resperpine." *Henry For Med. Bull.* 14 (June 1966), 109-118.

43 Chisholm, J., Jr. "Chelation therapy in children with subclinical plumbism." *Pediatrics* 53 (1974), 441.

44 Gordon, G., and Harper, H. Studies submitted to Food and Drug Administration, July, 1974. American Academy of Medical Preventics, North Hollywood, Calif.

45 Lamar, C. P. "Chelation therapy of occlusive arteriosclerosis in diabetic patients." *Angiology* 15 (1964), 379.

Chapter Six

1 Schroeder, H. A. *The Poisons Around Us*. Bloomington, Ind.: Indiana University Press, 1974.

2 Kopito, L., Brilet, A. M. and Schwachman, H. "Chronic plumbism in children: Diagnosis by hair analysis." *J.A.M.A.* 209 (1969), 243-248.

3 Vitale, L. P., et al. "Blood lead — An inadequate measure of occupational exposure." *J. Occup. Med.* 17:3 (1975), 155.

4 Seppalainen, A. M., et al. "Subclinical neuropathy at 'safe' levels of exposure." *Arch Environ. Health* (1975).

5 Graham, A., and Graham, F. "Lead poisoning and the suburban child." *Today's Health*, March, 1974.

6 Caprio, R. J.; Margulis, H. I.; and Joselow, M. "Lead absorption in children and its relationship to urban traffic densities." *Arch. Environ. Health* 28 (1975), 195-197.

7 Freeman, R. "Reversible myocarditis due to chronic lead poisoning in childhood." *Arch. Dis. Child.* 40 (1965), 389-393.

8 Strain, W. H., et al. (eds.) *Clinical Application of Zinc Metabolism*. Springfield, Ill.: Charles C. Thomas, Publisher, 1974.

[9] Isaacs, J. P., and Lamb, J. C. "Trace metals, vitamins, and hormones in ten-year treatment of coronary atherosclerotic heart disease." Library of Congress Catalog Card Number 74-82882, as delivered at the Texas Heart Institute Symposium on Coronary Artery Medicine and Surgery, Houston, February 21, 1974.

[10] Marsh, L. and Fraser, F. C. "Chelating agents and teratogenesis." *Lancet* (1973), 846.

[11] Perry, H. M., Jr., and Schroeder, H. A. "Lesions resembling vitamin B-complex deficiency and urinary loss of zinc produced by EDTA." *Am. J. Med. 22* (1957), 168-172.

[12] Foreman, H. "Toxic side effects of EDTA." *J. Chron. Dis. 16* (1963), 319-323.

[13] Perry, H. M., Jr. and Perry, E. F, "Normal concentrations of some trace metals in human urine, changes produced by EDTA." *J. Clin. Invest. 38* (1959), 1452.

[14] Tidball, C. S. "Nonspecificity of cation depletion when using chelators in biological systems." *Gastroenterology 60* (1971), 481.

[15] Davies, J. T. *The Clinical Significance of the Essential Biological Metals*. Springfield, Ill.: Charles C. Thomas, Publisher, 1972.

[16] Schettler, G., and Weizel, A. (eds.) *Atherosclerosis*. 111: *Proceedings of the Third International Symposium*. New York, Heidelberg, Berlin, Springer Verlag, 1974.

[17] Baumslag, N., et al. "Hair-metal binding." *Environ. Health Perspec. 8* (1974), 191-199.

[18] Hinners, T. A., et al. "Trace element nutriture and metabolism through head hair analysis." Department of Surgery, Case Western Reserve University School of Medicine, Cleveland.

[19] Hammer, D. I., et al. "Trace metals in human hair as a simple epidemiologic monitor of environmental exposure." National Environmental Research Center, Environmental Protection Agency, Research Triangle Park, N.C.

[20] Hoekstra, W. G., and Suttie, J. W. (eds.): *Trace Element Metabolism in Animals, II*. University Park Press, 1974.

[21] Kurliandchikov, V. N. "Treatment of patients with coronary arteriosclerosis with Unithiol in combination with decamevit." *Vrach. Delo. 6* (1974), 8.

[22] Zapadnick, V. I., et al. "Pharmacological activity of Unithiol and its use in clinical practice." *Vrach. Delo. 8* (1973), 122.

[23] Brucknerova, O., and Tulacek, J. "Chelates in the treatment of occlusive atherosclerosis." *Unitr. Lek. 18* (1972), 729.

[24] Levy, R. I., et al. "Dietary and drug treatment of primary hyperlipoproteinemia." *Ann. Intern. Med 77* (1972), 267.

[25] Popovici, A., et al. "Experimental control of serum calcium levels *in vivo*." Georgetown University Medical Center. *Proc. Soc. Ex. Biol. & Med. 74* (1950), 415-417.

[26] Rostenberg, A., Jr., and Perkins, A. J. "Nickel and cobalt dermatitis." *J. Allergy 22*: 466, 1951.

[27] Proescher, F. "Anticoagulant Properties of Ethylene-diamine tetra-acetic acid." *Proc. Soc. Exper. Biol. & Med. 76*: 619, 1951.

[28] Clarke, N. E.; Clarke, C. N.; and Mosher, R. D. "The *in vivo* dissolution of metastatic calcium: an approach to atherosclerosis." *Am. J. M. So. 229*: 142, 1955.

[29] Clarke, N. E.; Clarke, C. N.; and Mosher, R. E. "Treatment of angina pectoris with disodium-ethylene diamine tetraacetic acid." *Am. J. Med. Sci. 232* (1956), 654-666.

[30] Lamar, C. P. "Chelation therapy of occlusive arteriosclerosis in diabetic patients." *Angiology 15* (1964), 379.

[31] Lamar, C. P. "Calcium chelation of atherosclerosis — nine years' clinical experience." Fourteenth Annual Meeting, American College of Angiology, 1968.

[32] Oser, B., et al. "Safety evaluation studies of calcium EDTA." *Toxicol. Appl. Pharmacol. 5* (1963), 142-162.

[33] Doolan, P. D., et al. "An evaluation of the nephrotoxicity of ethylene diamine tetraacetate and diethylene triamine pentaacetate in the rat." *Toxicol. Appl. Pharmacol. 10* (1967), 481-500.
[34] Schwartz, S. L.; Johnson, C. B.; and Doolan, P. D. "Study of the mechanism of renal vacuologenesis induced in the rat by EDTA." *Mol. Pharmacol. 6* (1970), 54-60.
[35] Schwartz, S., et al. "Subcellular localization of EDTA in the proximal tubular cell of the rat kidney." *Biochem. Pharmacol. 16* (1967), 2413-2419.
[36] Seven, M. J. "Observations on the dosage of I.V. chelating agents." *Antibiot. MED. 5* (1958), 251.

Chapter Seven

[1] Cornfield, J., and Mitchell, S. "Selected risk factors in coronary disease." *Arch. Environ. Health 19* (1969), 382-294.
[2] Vavrik, M. "High risk factors and atherosclerotic cardiovascular diseases in the aged." *J. Am. Geriatr. Soc. 22* (1974), 203.
[3] Malmros, H. "Primary dietary prevention of atherosclerosis." *Bibl. Nutr. Dieta 19* (1973), 108.
[4] McGandy, R., et al. "Dietary fats, carbohydrates and atherosclerotic vascular disease." *N. Engl. J. Med. 277* (1967), 186.
[5] Moses, C. *Atherosclerosis: Mechanisms as a Guide to Prevention*. Philadelphia: Lea & Febiger, 1963.
[6] National Academy of Sciences, National Research Council. *Dietary Fat and Human Health*, Publ. No. 1147, 1966.
[7] Larsen, O. A., and Lassen, N. A. "Effects of daily muscular exercise in patients with intermittent claudication." *Lancet 2* (1966), 1093.
[8] Lamar, C. P. "Chelation therapy of occlusive arteriosclerosis in diabetic patients." *Angiology 15* (1964), 379.
[9] Lamar, C. P. "Calcium chelation of atherosclerosis — nine years' clinical experience." Fourteenth Annual Meeting, American College of Angiology, 1968.
[10] Passwater, Richard A. *Supernutrition*. New York: The Dial Press, 1975.
[11] Foreman, H.; Finnegan, C.; and Lushbaugh, C. C. "Nephrotoxic hazard from uncontrolled EDTA calcium-disodium therapy." *J.A.M.A. 160* (1956), 1042-1046.
[12] Dudley, H. R., and Ritchie, A. C. "Pathologic changes associated with the use of sodium EDTA in treatment of hypocalcemia." *N. Engl. J. Med. 252* (1955), 331-337.
[13] Seven, M. J. "Observations on the dosage of I.V. chelating agents." *Antibiot Med 5* (1958), 251.
[14] Doolan, P. D., et al. "An evaluation of the nephrotoxicity of ethylene diamine tetraacetate and diethylene triamine pentaacetate in the rat." *Toxicol. Appl. Pharacol. 10* (1967), 481-500.
[15] Schwartz, S. L.; Johnson, C. B.; and Doolan, P. D. "Study of the mechanism of renal vacuologenesis induced in the rate by EDTA." *Mol Pharacol. 6* (1970), 54-60.
[16] Schwartz, S. L., et al. "Subcellular localization of EDTA in the proximal tubular cell of the rat kidney." *Biochem Pharmacol. 16* (1967), 2413-2419.
[17] Oser, B., et al. "Safety evaluation studies of calcium EDTA." *Toxicol. Appl. Pharmacol. 5* (1963), 142-162.
[18] Meltzer, L. E.; Palmon, F., and Kitchell, J. R. "Long term use, side effects, and toxicity of disodium EDTA." *Am. J. Med. Sci. 242* (1961), 51-57.
[19] Sincock, A. "Life extension in the rotifer by application of chelating agents." *J. Gerontol. 30* (1975), 289-293.
[20] Foreman, H. "Toxic side effects of EDTA." *J. Chron. Dis. 16* (1963), 319-323.
[21] Perry, H. M., Jr., and Perry, E. F. "Normal concentrations of some trace metals in human urine, changes produced by EDTA." *J. Clin. Invest. 38* (1959), 1452.

[22] Tidball, C. S. "Nonspecifically of cation depletion when using chelators in biological systems." *Gastroenterology 60* (1971), 481.

[23] Perry, H. M., Jr., and Schroeder, H. A. "Lesions resembling vitamin B-complex deficiency and urinary loss of zinc produced by EDTA." *Am. J. Med.* 22 (1957), 168-172.

[24] Marsh, L., and Fraser, F. C. "Chelating agents and teratogenesis." *Lancet* 1973, 846.

[25] Matthew, H. *Side Effects of Drugs,* Volume VII. Amsterdam: Excerpta Medica, pp. 326-329.

Chapter Nine

[1] *Encyclopedia Americana* 25:186m, New York: Americana Corporation, 1966.

[2] *Pension Plan Guide, 1976 Social Security and Medicare Explained.* Chicago: Commerce Clearing House, Inc., 1976.

[3] Geha, A. S., et al. *J. Thorac. Cardiovasc. Surg.* 70:414, 1975.

[4] Loop, F. D., et al. *Am. J. Cardiol* 37:890, May 1976.

[5] Tecklenberg, P. L., et al. *Circulation 52*, Suppl. I:98, 1975.

[6] Winkle, R. A., et al. *Circulation 52*, Suppl. I:61, 1975.

Chapter Ten

[1] Mundth, E. D., and Austen, W. G. *N. Engl. J. Med. 293:13*, 75, 124, 1975.

[2] "Coronary arteriography and coronary artery surgery." *The Medical Letter 18*, 14 (issue 456), July 2, 1976.

[3] Adams, D. F., et al. *Circulation 48*:609, 1973.

[4] Zir, L. M., et al. *Circulation 53*:627, April, 1976.

[5] Millman, Marcia. *The Unkindest Cut: Life in the Backrooms of Medicine.* New York: William Morrow and Co., Inc., 1977.

[6] Brody, Jane E. "Doctors query bypass surgery as aid to heart." *The New York Times.* Nov. 22, 1976.

[7] Geha, A. S., et al. *J. Thorac. Cardiovasc. Surg.* 70:414, 1975.

[8] Loop, F. D., et al. *Am. J. Cardiol* 37:890, May, 1976.

[9] Tecklenberg, P. L., et al. *Circulation 52, Suppl 1*:61, 1975.

[10] Winkle, R. A., et al. *Circulation, 52, Suppl 1*:61, 1975.

[11] Berg, Jr., R., et al. *J. Thorac. Cardiovasc. Surg.* 70:432, 1975.

[12] Winterscherd, L. C., et al. *Amer. Surg.* 41:520, Sept. 1975.

[13] Keon, W. J., et al. *Can. Med. Assoc. J.* 114: 312, Feb. 21, 1976.

[14] Alderman, E. L., et al. *N. Engl. J. Med. 288*: 535, 1973.

[15] Bassan, M. M., et al. *N. Engl. J. Med. 290*: 349, 1974.

[16] Cohen, M. V., and Gorlin, R. *Circulation 52*: 275, 1975.

[17] Takan, T., et al. *Circulation 52, Suppl. II*: 143, 1975.

[18] Selden, R., et al. *N. Engl. J. Med. 293*: 1329, 1975.

[19] Mathur, V. S., and Guinin, G. A. *Circulation, 52, Suppl. I*: 133, 1975.

[20] Kloster, F., et al. *Circulation, 52, Suppl. II*: 90, 1975.

[21] Russell, R. D., et al. *Am. J. Cardiol. 37*: 896, May, 1976.

[22] "Heart bypasses are often unnecessary, study says." *The New York Times,* March 10, 1977.

[23] "Bypass blocked — but still no angina." *Medical World News,* Aug. 9, 1976, p. 68.

[24] "Comparing treatments for angina." *Medical World News,* April 7, 1975.

[25] Kansal, S., et al. "Ischemic myocardial injury following aortocoronary bypass surgery." *Chest 67* (1975), 20-26.

[26] Kouchoukas, N. T., et al. "An appraisal of coronary bypass grafting." *Circulation 50* (1974), 11.

[27] Kouchoukas, N. T., "Operative therapy for femoropopliteal arterial occlusive disease — A comparison of therapeutic methods." *Circulation (Suppls.) 35* (1967), 1-178, *36* (1967), 1-182.
[28] Thompson, J. E., "Acute peripheral arterial occlusions." *N. Engl. J. Med. 290* (1974), 950.
[29] Segal, B. L., et al. "Saphenous vein bypass surgery for coronary artery disease." *Am. J. Cardiol. 32* (1973), 1010-1013.
[30] Mundth, E. D., and Austen, W. G. "Surgical Measures for coronary heart disease." *N. Engl. J. Med. 293* (1975), 124-129.
[31] Fulton, R. L., and Blakely, W. R., "Lumbar sympathectomy: A procedure of questionable value in the treatment of arteriosclerosis obliteraus of the legs." *Am. J. Surg. 116* (1968), 735.

Chapter Eleven
[1] Nikitina, E. K. "Treatment of arterosclerosis with Trilon B (EDTA)." *Kardiologia 12* (11): 137, Nov. 1972.
[2] Zapadnick, V. I. et al. "Pharmacological activity of Unithiol and its use in clinical practice." *Vrach Delo. 8:* 122, 1973.
[3] Kurliandchikov, V. N. "Treatment of patients with coronary arteriosclerosis with Unithiol in combination with Decamevit." *Vrach. Delo. 6:* 8, 1973.

Chapter Twelve
[1] Meltzer, L. E.; Palmon, F.; and Kitchell, J. R. "Long term use, side effects, and toxicity of disodium EDTA." *Am. J. Med. Sci. 242* (1961), 51-57.
[2] "Peripheral flow opened up." *Medical World News*, March 15, 1963, pp. 37-39.
[3] Kitchell, J. R., et al. "The treatment of coronary artery disease with disodium EDTA — A reappraisal." *Am. J. Cardiol. 11* (1963), 501-506.
[4] Kitchell, J. R.; Meltzer, L. E.; and Rutman, E. "Effects of ions on *in vitro* gluconeogenesis in rat kidney cortex slices." *Am. J. Physiol. 208* (1965), 841-846.
[5] Clarke, N. E.; Clarke, C. N.; and Mosher, R. E. "Treatment of angina pectoris with disodium ethylene diamine tetraacetic acid." *Am. J. Med. Sci. 232* (1965), 654-666.
[6] Clarke, N. E., Sr., Clarke, N. E., Jr., and Moser, R. E. "Treatment of occlusive vascular disease with disodium ethylene diamine tetraacetic acid (EDTA)." *Am. J. Med. Sci. 239* (1960), 732-744.
[7] Kitchell, J. R.; Meltzer, L. E.; and Seven, M. J. "Potential uses of chelation methods in the treatment of cardiovascular disease." *Prog. Cardiovasc. Dis. 19* (1961), 798.
[8] Seven, M. J. (ed.). *Metal Binding in Medicine*. Philadelphia: J. B. Lippincott Company, 1960.
[9] Seven, M. J., and Johnson, L. "Proceedings of a conference on biological aspects of metal binding." *Fed. Proc.* (Suppl. 10, 1961).
[10] Brucknerova, O. and Tulacek, J. "Chelates in the treatment of occlusive atherosclerosis," *Vnitr. Lek. 18* (1972), 729.
[11] Kurliandchikov, V. N. "Treatments of patients with coronary arteriosclerosis with Unithiol in combination with Decamevit." *Vrach, Delo. 6.* (1973), 8.
[12] Ohno, T. "Clinical and experimental studies of arteriosclerosis." *Excerpta Medica: Intern, Med. 17:* 8 (1963).
[13] Meltzer, L. E.; Urol, M. E.; and Kitchell, J. R. "The treatment of coronary artery disease with disodium EDTA." In Seven, M. J. (ed.). *Metal Binding in Medicine*. Philadelphia: J. B. Lippincott Co., 1960, pp. 132-136.

Chapter Thirteen

[1] "Palm Desert Man Tells Meadowbrook Experience." *National Health Federation Bulletin* XXI: 6-9, October, 1975.
[2] "Louisiana." *Encyclopedia Americana* 17:784, New York: Americana Corporation, 1966.
[3] "New Warning on Therapy." *Salt Lake Tribune*, August 22, 1976.
[4] National Educational Society for Natural Healing, Post Office Box 15758, New Orleans, Louisiana 70175.

Chapter Fourteen

[1] Soffer, A. "Chelation treatment for arteriosclerosis." *JAMA 233* (1975).
[2] Craven, P. C., and Morelli, H. F. "Chelation therapy." *West. J. Med. 122* (1975), 277-278.
[3] "CMA warns against chelation." *CMA News 20*: 13, Sept. 12, 1975, p. 3.
[4] Kannel, W. "Long-term value of coronary bypass disputed." *Family Practice News* 6:1.
[5] Petersdorf, R. G. "Internal medicine in family practice." *N. Engl. J. Med. 293* (1975), 326.
[6] Kaegor, Bill. "Probation urged for physician." *Today*, Dec. 18, 1976.
[7] Wolinsky, Howard. "Treatment under attack." *Today*, Jan. 10, 1977.

Chapter Fifteen

[1] Soffer, Alfred. "Chihuahuas and laetrile, chelation therapy, and honey from Boulder, Colo." *Arch. Intern. Med 136*: 865 & 866, Aug. 1976.
[2] Kell, George W. Brief filed with Curtis L. Klahs in the matter of Ophelia Clementino, Sept. 9, 1976.
[3] Kell, George W. Brief filed with Curtis L. Klahs in the matter of Ophelia Clementino, Sept. 3, 1976.
[4] In the Matter of Ophelia V. Clementino, HIC #236-03-7068-B, "Decision of Hearing Officer." *Proceedings before the Occidental Life Insurance Company of California*, Sept. 13, 1976.
[5] Turk, Randall. "San Gabriel man is living, active testament to alternative therapy." *Star-News*, Pasadena, CA, June 21, 1976.

Appendix

Suggested General References from the Medical, Nutritional and Laboratory Literature by Subject

Cardiovascular System

Arrhythmias

The effect of Na₃EDTA-induced hypocalcemia upon the general and coronary hemodynamics of the intact animal. (MAXWELL, G. M., Elliott, R. B. and Robertson, E.) *Am Heart J* 66:82-87, 1963. (13)

Rate of rise of left ventricular pressure. Indirect measurement and physiologic significance. (LANDRY, JR., A. B. and Goodyer, A. V. N.) *Am J. Cardiol* 15:660-664, 1965. (22)

Quinidine toxicity and its treatment. An experimental study. (LUCHI, R. J., Helwig, Jr., J. and Conn, Jr., H. L.) *Am Heart J* 65:340-348, 1963. (20)

Intensification of the effects of quinidine on experimental auricular fibrillation in the dog previously treated with the disodium salt of ethylene diamine tetraacetate. (BOYADJIAN, N.) *C R Soc Biol* 155:414-416, 1961. (6)

Ventricular arrhythmias following the administration of Na₂EDTA. (NAYLER, W. G.) *Pharmacol Exp Ther* 137:5-13, 1962. (24)

Treatment of cardiac arrhythmias with salts of ethylene diamine tetraacetic acid (EDTA). (SURAWICZ, B., MacDonald, M. G., Kaljot, V., Bettinger, J C., Carpenter, A. A., Korson, L. and Starcheska, Y. K.) *Am Heart J* 58:493-503, 1959. (32)

Myocardial responses to chelation. (SOFFER, A., Toribara, T. and Sayman, A.) *Brit Heart J* 23:690-694, 1961. (20)

Clinical applications and untoward reactions of chelation in cardiac arrhythmias. (SOFFER, A., Toribara, T., Moore-Jones, C. and Weber, D.) *AMA Arch Intern Med* 106:824-834, 1960. (18)

The effect of calcium chelation on cardiac arrhythmias and conduction disturbances. (JICK, S. and Karsh, R.) *Am J Cardiol* 4:287-293, 1959. (18)

Effects of pacemaker impulses on latent arrhythmias produced by intramyocardial chemical stimulation. (CASTELLANOS, JR., A., Lemberg, L., Gomez, A. and Berkovits, B. V.) *Cardiologia* 51:340-348, 1967. (15)

Arteries (Animal)

Effect of copper in thyroxine potentiation of in vitro epinephrine action on smooth muscle. (SHIDA, H., Meyers, M. A. and Barker, S. B.) *J Pharmacol Exp Ther* 141:280-284, 1963. (14)

Role of calcium in initiation of contraction in smooth muscle. (ISOJIMA, C. and Bozler, E.) *Am J Physiol* 205:681-685, 1963. (25)

Influence of ethylene diamine tetraacetate and calcium ions on vascular tension. (LASZT, L.) *Nature 212*:1587, 1966. (18)

Sucrose-gap recording of prolonged electrical activity from arteries in Ca-free solution containing EDTA at low temperature. (GRAHAM, J. M. and Keatinge, W. R.) *J Physiol 208*:2P-3P, 1970. (3)

Responsiveness of arterial smooth muscle to noradrenaline after long periods of Ca-free solution containing EDTA at low temperature. (KEATINGE, W. R.) *J Physiol 216*:31P, 1971. (3)

Effect of EDTA and other chelating agents on norepinephrine uptake by rabbit aorta in vitro. (NEDERGAARD, O. A. and Vagne, A.) *Proc West Pharmacol Soc 11*:87-90, 1968. (3)

Arteriosclerosis
Chelates in the treatment of occlusive arteriosclerosis. (BRUCKNEROVA, O. and Tulacek, J.) *Vnitr Lek 18*:729-736, 1972. (25)

1st experience with the treatment of atherosclerosis patients with calcinosis of the arteries with trilon B (disodium salt of EDTA). (ARONOV, D. M.) *Klin Med (Moskva) 41*:19-23, May 1963. (15)

Atherosclerosis, occlusive vascular disease and EDTA. (Ed) (CLARKE, SR., N. E.) *Am J Cardiol 6*:233-236, 1960. (18)

The treatment of coronary artery disease with disodium EDTA. A reappraisal. (KITCHELL, J. R., Palmon, Jr., F., Aytan, N. and Meltzer, L. E.) *Am J Cardiol 11*:501-506, 1963. (7)

Chelation endarterectomy for occlusive atherosclerosis. (LAMAR, C. P.) *J Am Geriat Soc 14*:272-294, 1966. (28)

Arteriosclerosis therapy with mucopolysaccharides and EDTA. (FRIEDEL, W., Schulz, F. H. and Schroder, I.) *Deutsch Gesundh 20*:1566-1570, 1965. (37)

Reduction of elevated plasma lipid levels in atherosclerosis following EDTA therapy. (OLWIN, J. H. and Koppel, J. L.) *Proc Soc Exp Biol Med 128*:1137-1140, 1968. (5)

Treatment of occlusive vascular disease with disodium ethylene diamine tetraacetic acid (EDTA). (CLARKE, SR., N. E., Clarke, Jr. N. E. and Mosher, R. E.) *Am J Med Sci 239*:732-744, 1960. (50)

Depression of cholesterol levels in human plasma following ethylene diamine tetraacetate and hydralazine. (PERRY, JR., H. M. and Schroeder, H. A.) *J Chron Dis 2*:520-533, 1955. (20)

The effects of chelating agents upon the atherosclerotic process. (ANONYMOUS) *Nutr Rev 21*:352, 1963. (3)

Mobilization of atherosclerotic plaque calcium with EDTA utilizing the isolation-perfusion principle. (WILDER, L. W., De Jode, L. R., Milstein, S. W. and Howard, J. M.) *Surgery 52*:793-795, 1962. (6)

Arteriosclerosis (Animal)
Effect of calcium disodium ethylene diamine tetraacetate on hypercholesterolemic rabbits. (SAUNDERS, J. F., Princiotto, J. V. and Rubin, M.) *Proc Soc Exp Biol Med 92*:29-31, 1956. (9)

Effect of chelation on phosphorus metabolism in experimental atherosclerosis. (McCANN, D. S., Koen, Z., Zdybek, G. and Boyle, A. J.) *Circ Res 11*:880-884, 1962. (7)

Some in vivo effects of chelation. II. Animal experimentation. (KOEN, A., McCann, D. S. and Boyle, A. J.) *J Chron Dis 16*:329-333, 1963. (8)

Physical and chemical changes in isolated chylomicrons: prevention by EDTA. (ONTKA, J. A.) *J Lipid Res 11*:367-375, 1970. (32)

Blood
Changes in hematologic values induced by storage of ethylene diamine tetraacetate human blood for varying periods of time. (LAMPASSO, J. A.) *Am J Clin Path 49*:443-447, 1968. (11)

Failure of anticoagulants to influence the viscosity of whole blood. (GALLUZZI, N. J., DeLashmutt, R. E. and Connolly, V. J.) *J Lab Clin Med 64*:773-777, 1964. (7)

Investigation on the influence of diamethylsulfoxide on conservation of the whole blood at low temperatures. (FIDELSKI, R., Niedworok, J. and Pniewski, T.) *Bibl Haemat 23*:667-673, 1965. (22)

Comparative effects of anticoagulants on bacterial growth in experimental blood cultures. (EVANS, G. L., Cekoric, Jr., T. and Searcy, R. L.) *Am J Med Techn 34*:103-112, 1968. (20)

Studies on the origin and significance of blood ammonia. I. Effect of various anticoagulants on the blood ammonia determination. (CONN, H. O.) *Yale J Biol Med 35*:171-184, 1962. (35)

Blood (Animal)
Effect of manganese edetate on blood formation in rats. (SULLIVAN, T. J.) *Nature 186*:87, 1960. (5)

The effect of heparin and EDTA on DNA synthesis by marrow in vitro. (LOCHTE, JR., H. L., Ferrebee, J. W. and Thomas, E. D.) *J Lab Clin Med 55*:435-438, 1960. (11)

Blood Clotting
The effect of EDTA on human fibrinogen and its significance for the coagulation of fibrinogen with thrombin. (GODAL, H. C.) *Scand J Clin Lab Invest 12* (Suppl 53):1-20, 1960. (32)

Barium sulphate adsorption and elution of the 'prothrombin complex' factors. (VOSS, D.) *Scand J Clin Lab Invest 17* (Suppl 84):119-128, 1965. (19)

The precipitation of fibrinogen by heparin at pH 4.8. (TEMPERLEY, I. J.) *Irish J Med Sci 448*:159-166, 1963. (14)

Role of calcium in the structure of fibrinogen. (CAPET-ANTONINI, F. C.) *Biochim Biophys Acta 200*:497-507, 1970. (17)

Effect of various anticoagulants on carbon dioxide-combining power of blood. (ZARODA, R. A.) *AM J Clin Path 41*:377-380, 1964. (8)

Delayed fibrin polymerization due to removal of calcium ions. (GODAL, H. C.) *Scand J Clin Lab Invest 24*:29-33, 1969. (15)

Blood Erythrocytes

Oxidation of hemoglobin by ethylene diamine tetraacetate and leukocytes. (NORDQVIST, P., Persson, E., Ryttinger, L. and Ljunggren, M.) *Scand J Clin Lab Invest* 15:62-66, 1963. (5)

Observations on the hexokinase activity in intact human erythrocytes. (GARBY, L. and De Verdier, C. H.) *Folia Haemat* 83:313-316, 1965. (11)

Effects of ethylene diamine tetraacetate and deoxycholate on kinetic constants of the calcium ion-dependent adenosine triphosphatase of human erythrocyte membranes. (WOLF, H. U.) *Biochem J* 130:311-314, 1972. (15)

The effect of the anticoagulant EDTA on oxygen uptake by bone-marrow cells. (GESINSKI, R. M. and Morrison, J. H.) *Experientia* 24:296-297, 1968. (8)

Hemorrhagic and hemolytic transfusion reaction due to anti-Lea . (MACPHERSON, C. R., Teteris, N. J. and Claassen, L. G.) *Transfusion* 3:392-396, 1963. (12)

Sedimentation rate of stored blood, using sequestrene as the anticoagulant. (MELVILLE, I. D. and Rifkind, B. M.) *Brit Med J* 1:107-109, 1960. (2)

Error in hematocrit value produced by excessive ethylene diamine tetraacetate. (LAMPASSO, J. A.) *Techn Bull Regist Med Techn* 35:109-110, 1965. (2)

Elimination of error in hematocrit produced by excessive EDTA. Experience with the Coulter Counter Model S. (BRITTIN, G. M., Brecher, G. and Johnson, C. A.) *Techn Bull Regist Med Techn* 39:246-249, 1969. (3)

The effect of anticoagulant concentration on centrifuged and electronic hematocrits. (FERRO, P. V. and Sena, T.) *Am J Clin Path* 51:569-577, 1969. (9)

Error in hematocrit determination due to too high concentration of anticoagulant. (CULLUM, C. and Lepow, M. L.) *Pediatrics* 40:1027-1028, 1967. (3)

The Westergren sedimentation rate, using K₃EDTA. (GAMBINO, S. R., Di Re, J. J., Montellone, M. and Budd, D. C.) *Techn Bull Regist Med Techn* 35:1-8, 1965. (7)

Effect of ethylene diamine tetraacetic acid (dipotassium salt) and heparin on the estimation of packed cell volume. (PENNOCK, C. A. and Jones, K. W.) *J Clin Path* 19:196-199, 1966. (12)

The inhibitory action of EDTA on erythrocyte agglutination by lectins. (TUNIS, M.) *J Immun* 95:876-879, 1965. (15)

Separation of haemoglobins Lepore and H from A and A₂ in starch or acrylamide gels buffered with tris-EDTA. (CURTAIN, C. C.) *J Clin Path* 15:288-289, 1962. (7)

Error in hematocrit value produced by excessive ethylene diamine tetraacetate. (LAMPASSO, J. A.) *Am J Clin Path* 44:109-110, 1965. (2)

5-Year controlled trial of chelating agents in treatment of thalassaemia major. (FLYNN, D. M.) *Arch Dis Child* 48:829, 1973. (0)

A serum agglutinating human red cells exposed to EDTA. (GILLUND, T. D., Howard, P. L. and Isham, B.) *Vox Sang* 23:369-370, 1972. (4)

Study of human red blood cell membrane using sodium deoxycholate. II. Effects of cold storage, EDTA and small deoxycholate concentrations on ATPase activities. (PHILPPOT, J. and Authier, M. H.) *Biochim Biophys Acta* 298:887-900, 1973. (32)

Blood Erythrocytes (Animal)
The effects of metallic edetates on the growth and blood formation of rats. (SULLI-VAN, T. J.) *Arch Int Pharmacodyn 124*:225-236, 1960. (21)

The inhibition of hematopoietic action of iron by ethylene diamine tetraacetic acid (EDTA). (ITOH, H., Yamaguchi, T. and Yamasawa, S.) *Yokohama Med Bull 13*:9-16, 1962. (6)

Blood Leukocytes
Pathogenesis of acute inflammation, VI. Influence of osmolarity and certain metabolic antagonists upon phagocytosis and adhesiveness by leucocytes recovered from man. (ALLISON, JR., F. and Lancaster, M. G.) *Proc Soc Exp Biol Med 119*:56-61, 1965. (13)

Studies on factors which influence the adhesiveness of leukocytes in vitro. (ALLISON, JR., F. and Lancaster, M. G.) *Ann NY Acad Sci 116*:936-944, 1964. (6)

The action in vitro and in vivo of sodium versenate on the phagocytic activity of neutrophile leukocytes. (FORSSMAN, O. and Nordqvist, P.) *Acta Haemat 31*:289-293, 1964. (9)

The relationship between phagocytosis of polystyrene latex particles by polymor-phonuclear leucocytes (PML) and aggregation of PML. (TALSTAD, I.) *Scand J Haemat 9*:516-523, 1972. (15)

The prevention of clumping of frozen-stored leukocyte populations by EDTA. (BOCK, G. N., Chess, L. and Mardinay, Jr., M. R.) *Cryobiology 9*:216-218, 1972. (9)

EDTA-Na2 and leukocytes. (KISSMEYER-NIELSEN, F. and Andresen, E.) *Bibl Haemat 19*:434-438, 1964. (1)

Rapid collection of human leukocytes or lymphocytes from peripheral blood. (SEVERSON, C. D., Frank, D. H., Stokes, G., Seepersad, M. F. and Thompson, J. S.) *Transplantation 8*:535-538, 1969. (8)

Histochemical studies on leucocyte alkaline phosphatase in non-leukaemic granulocytosis: effects of anticoagulants and role of zinc and magnesium. (PERILLIE, P. E. and Finch, S. C.) *Brit J Haemat 13*:289-293, 1967. (6)

Isolation of leococytes from human blood. Further observations. Methylcellulose, dextran, and ficoll as erythrocyte-aggrevating agents. (BOYUM, A.) *Scand J Clin Lab Invest 21* (Supl 97):31-50, 1968. (21)

The technique and interpretation of tests for leucocidin with special reference to the value of ethylene diamine tetraacetic acid (EDTA). (McLEOD, J. A. and McLeod, J. W.) *Brit J Exp Path 42*:171-178, 1961. (12)

Blood Plasma
Cholesterol measurement in serum and plasma. (GRANDE, F., Amatuzio, D. S. and Wada, S.) *Clin Chem 10*:619-626, 1964. (15)

Measurement of renin activity in human plasma. (PICKENS, P. T., Bumpus, F. M., Lloyd, A. M., Smeby, R. R. and Page, I. H.) *Circ Res 17*:438-448, 1965. (19)

Serum-insulin or plasma-insulin? (Letters) (GRANT, D. B.) *Lancet 1*:207, 1972. (0)

The distribution of EDTA and citrate in blood and plasma. (REUTER, H., Niemeyer, G. and Gross, R.) *Thromb Diath Haemorrh 19*:213-220, 1968. (3)

200 CHELATION THERAPY

Binding of EDTA, histidine and acetylsalicylic acid to zinc-protein complex in intestinal content, intestinal mucosa and blood plasma. (SUSO, F. A. and Edwards, Jr.,
H. M.) *Nature* 236:230-232, 1972. (10)

Change in plasma phosphate concentration on infusion of calcium gluconate or
Na₂-EDTA. (HAUSMANN, E.) *Proc Soc Exp Biol Med* 134:182-184, 1970. (12)

Blood Platelets
Pseudothrombocytopenia: manifestation of a new type of platelet agglutinin.
(SHREINER, D. P. and Bell, W. R.) *Blood* 42:531-549, 1973. (20)

Influence of cryoprofibrin on the antiglobulin consumption test with platelets. (VAN
DER WEERDT, C. M. and Vreeken, J.) *Vox Sang* 10:536-542, 1965. (3)

Release reaction in washed platelet suspensions induced by kaolin and other particles. (CRONBERG, S. and Caen, J. P.) *Scand J Haemat* 8:151-160, 1971. (24)

Effects of ethylene diamine tetraacetate (EDTA) and citrate upon platelet glycolysis.
(ROSSI, E. C.) *J Lab Clin Med* 69:204-216, 1967. (24)

Studies on the ultrastructure of pseudopod formation in human blood platelets. I.
Effect of temperature, period of incubation, anticoagulants and mechanical forces.
(SKJORTEN, F.) *Scand J Haemat* 5:401-414, 1968. (11)

Effect of aggregating agents and their inhibitors on the mean platelet shape.
(O'BRIEN, J. R. and Heywood, J. B.) *J Clin Path* 19:148-153, 1966. (5)

Platelet sequestration in man. I. Methods. (ASTER, R. H. and Jandl, J. H.) *J Clin Invest*
43:843-855, 1964. (44)

Effect of glass contact on the electrophoretic mobility of human blood platelets.
(HAMPTON, J. R. and Mitchell, J. R. A.) *Nature* 209:470-472, 1966. (7)

The role of chelation and of human plasma in the uptake of serotonin by human
platelets. (KERBY, G. P. and Taylor, S. M.) *J Clin Invest* 40:44-51, 1961. (15)

The evaluation of anticoagulant solutions used in the preparation of platelets for
transfusion. (DAVEY, M. G., Lander, H. and Robson, H. N.) *Bibl Haemat* 23:1358-
1361, 1965. (6)

Platelet preservation. III. Comparison of radioactivity yields of platelet concentrates
derived from blood anticoagulated with EDTA and ACD. (COHEN, P., Cooley,
M. H. and Gardner, F. H.) *New Eng J Med* 273:845-850, 1965. (16)

Evaluation of a technic for counting dog and human platelets. (WEED, R. I., Crump,
S. L., Swisher, S. N. and Trabold, N. C.) *Blood* 25:261-266, 1965. (8)

Platelet aggregation by ristocetin in EDTA plasma: extensive clumping with high
concentrations of EDTA. (TS'AO, C. H.) *Haemostasis* 1:315-319, 1972/73. (5)

A macromolecular serum component acting on platelets in the presence of EDTA —
'platelet stain preventing factor.' (STAVEM, P. and Berg, K.) *Scand J Haemat* 10:202-
208, 1973. (2)

Effects of ethylene diamine tetraacetic acid (EDTA) on platelet structure. (WHITE,
J. G.) *Scand J Haemat* 5:241-254, 1968. (23)

Blood Pressure
Renal and cardiovascular effects induced by intravenous infusion of magnesium
chelates. (KELLEY, H. G., Turton, M. R. and Hatcher, J. D.) *Canad Med Assoc J*
84:1124-1128, 1961. (6)

Blood Pressure (Animal)

Action of a chelate of zinc on trace metals in hypertensive rats. (SCHROEDER, H. A., Nason, A. P. and Mitchener, M.) *Am J Physiol 214*:796-800, 1968. (13)

Antihypertensive effects of metal binding agents. (SCHROEDER, H. A., Perry, Jr., H. M., Menhard, E. M. and Dennis, E. G.) *J Lab Clin Med 46*:416-422, 1955. (12)

On the cardiovascular activities of the sodium salt of ethylene diamine tetraacetic acid. (MARCELLE, R. and L'eComte, J.) *C R Soc Biol 153*:1483-1485, 1959. (1)

Blood Serum

Changes in serum and spinal fluid calcium effected by disodium ethylene diamine tetraacetate. (SOFFER, A. and Toribara, T.) *J Lab Clin Med 58*:542-547, 1961. (10)

The binding of EDTA to human serum albumin. (ANGHILERI, L. J.) *Naturwissenschaften 55*:182, 1968. (0)

Serum calcium and phosphorus homeostatis in man studied by means of the sodium-EDTA test. (KALLIOMAKI, J. L., Markkanen, T. K. and Mustonen, V. A.) *Acta Med Scand 170*:211-214, 1961. (9)

Determination of calcium in solutions containing ethylene diamine tetraacetic acid. (TORIBARA, T. Y. and Koval, L.) *J Lab Clin Med 57*:630-634, 1961. (6)

Semimicro method for determination of serum uric acid using EDTA-hydrazine. (PATEL, C. P.) *Clin Chem 14*:764-775, 1968. (10)

Digitalis

Effects of calcium chelation on digitalis-induced cardiac arrhythmias. (SZEKELY. P. and Wynne, N. A.) *Brit Heart J 25*:589-594, 1963. (25)

The effect of disodium EDTA on digitalis intoxication. (ROSENBAUM, J. L., Mason, D. and Seven, M. J.) *Am J Med Sci 240*:77-84, 1960. (14)

Use of the chelating agent, EDTA, in digitalis intoxication and cardiac arrhythmias. (SURAWICZ, B.) *Progr Cardiov Dis 2*:432-443, 1960. (40)

Antagonism of the contractile effect of digitalis by EDTA in the normal human ventricle. (COHEN, S., Weissler, A. M. and Schoenfeld, C. D.) *Am Heart J 69*:502-514, 1965. (20)

Calcium, chelates, and digitalis. A clinical study. (ELIOT, R. S. and Blount, Jr., S. G.) *Am Heart J 62*:7-21, 1961. (15)

Treatment of digitalis intoxication with EDTA Na$_2$. (NGUYEN-THE-MINH) *Presse Med 71*:2385-2386, 1963. (5)

Lymph

Interaction of lymphocytes and phytohaemagglutinin: inhibition by chelating agents. (KAY, J. E.) *Exp Cell Res 68*:11-16, 1971. (25)

'Radial segmentation' of the nuclei in lymphocytes and other blood cells induced by some anticoagulants. (NORBERG, B. and Soderstrom, N.) *Scand J Haemat 4*:68-76, 1967. (11)

Veins

Topical chelation therapy for varicose pigmentation. (MYERS, H. L.) *Angiology 17*:66-68, 1966. (8) •

Dentistry

Human Studies
Scanning electron microscope studies of dental enamel. (HOFFMAN, S., McEwan, W. S. and Drew, C. M.) *J DentRes 48*:242-250, 1969. (15)

Disodium ethylene diamine tetraacetate as an aid for the reconstitution of lyophilized human salivary proteins before paper electrophoresis. (DAWES, C.) *Arch Oral Biol 8*:653-656, 1963. (10)

Differences in the shape of human enamel crystallites after partial destruction by caries, EDTA and various acids. (JOHNSON, N. W.) *Arch Oral Biol 11*:1421-1424, 1966. (25)

The relative efficiency of EDTA, sulfuric acid, and mechanical instrumentation in the enlargement of root canals. (WEINREB, M. M. and Meier, E.) *Oral Surg 19*:247-252, 1965. (18)

The effects of different demineralizing agents on human enamel surfaces studied by scanning electron microscopy. (POOLE, D. F. G. and Johnson, N. W.) *Arch Oral Biol 12*:1621-1634, 1967. (38)

In vivo and in vitro studies of the effect of the disodium salt of ethylene diamine tetraacetate on human dentine and its endodontic implications. (PATTERSON, S. S.) *Oral Surg 16*:83-103, 1963. (14)

An in vitro comparison of the amount of calcium removed by the disodium salt of EDTA and hydrochloric acid during endodontic procedures. (HELING, B., Shapiro, S. and Sciaky, I.) *Oral Surg 19*:531-533, 1965. (6)

The pharmacokinetics of fluoride in mouth rinses as indicated by a reference substance (^{51}Cr-EDTA). (BIRKELAND, J. M. and Lokken, P.) *Caries Res 6*:325-333, 1972. (19)

The solubility rate of calcified dental tissues and of calculus in sodium EDTA solutions. (SHAPIRO, S., Perez, G., Gedalia, I. and Sulman, F. G.) *J Periodont 39*:9-10, 1968.

Enamel conditioning for fluoride treatments. (KATZ, S., Muhler, J. C. and Beck, C. W.) *J Dent Res 50*:816-831, 1971. (36)

Solubility of calcified dental tissue and of calculus in EDTA and 2% NaF. (SHILOAH, J., Gedalia, I., Shapiro, S. and Jacobowitz, B.) *J Dent Res 52*:845, 1973. (7)

Two-site model for human dental enamel dissolution in EDTA. (FOX, J. L., Higuchi, W. I., Fawzi, M., Hwu, R. C. and Hefferren, J. J.) *J Dent Res 53*:939, 1974. (4)

The dissociation of EDTA and EDTA-sodium salts. (SAND, H. F.) *Acta Odont Scand 19*:469-482, 1961. (6)

Dermatology

Allergies
Nickel sensitization and detergents. (MALTEN, K. E., Schutter, K., Van Senden, K. G. and Spruit, D.) *Acta Dermatovener 49*:10-13, 1969. (7)

The relative importance of various environmental exposures to nickel in causing contact hypersensitivity. (MALTEN, K. E. and Spruit, D.) *Acta Dermatovener 49*:14-19, 1969. (22)

EDTA: preservative dermatitis. (RAYMOND, J. Z. and Gross, P. R.) *Arch Derm* 100:436-440, 1969. (12)

Burns (Animal)
Combinations of edetic acid and antibiotics in the treatment of rat burns infection with *Pseudomonas aeruginosa*. (WEISER, R.) *J Infect Dis* 128:566-569, 1973. (16)

Porphyria
Acute intermittent porphyria. (RITOTA, M. C. and Sanowski, R.) *J Med Soc New Jersey* 61:101-103, March 1964. (13)

Hexachlorobenzene-induced porphyria: effect of chelation on the disease, porphyrin and metal metabolism. (PETERS, H. A., Johnson, S. A. M., Cam, S., Oral, S., Muftu, Y. and Ergene, T.) *Am J Med Sci* 251:314-322, 1966. (44)

Current concepts of cutaneous porphyria and its treatment with particular reference to the use of sodium calciumedetate. (DONALD, G. F., Hunter, G. A., Roman, W. and Taylor, A. E. J.) *Brit J Derm* 82:70-75, 1970. (24)

Chelation therapy in cutaneous porphyria. A review and report of a five-year recovery. (WOODS, S. M., Peters, H. A. and Johnson, S. A. M.) *Arch Derm* 84:920-927, 1961. (28)

Porphyria. Its manifestations and treatment with chelating agents. (PAINTER, J. T. and Morrow, E. J.) *Texas State J Med* 55:811-818, 1959. (15)

Sclerosis
Use of the chelating agent edathamil disodium in acrosclerosis, sarcoidosis and other skin conditions with comments on tryptophan metabolism in sarcoidosis. (JOHNSON, S. A. M.) *Wisconsin Med J* 59:651-655, 1960. (0)

Use of ethylene diamine tetraacetic acid (EDTA) and tetrahydroxyquinone on sclerodermatous skin. Histologic and chemical studies. (KEECH, M. K., McCann, D. S., Boyle, A. J. and Pinkus, H.) *J Invest Derm* 47:235-246, 1966. (66)

Calcinosis universalis complicating dermatomyositis — its treatment with Na2EDTA. Report of two cases in children. (HERD, J. K. and Vaughan, J. H.) *Arthritis Rheum* 7:259-271, 1964. (53)

Treatment of calcinosis universalis with chelating agents. (FINK, C. W. and Baum, J.) *Am J Dis Child* 105:390-392, 1963. (5)

Edathamil (EDTA) therapy of interstitial calcinosis. (LECKERT, J. T., McHardy, G. G. and McHardy, R. J.) *South Med J* 53:728-731, 1960. (10)

The treatment of progressive systemic sclerosis with disodium edetate. (MONGAN, E. S.) *Arthritis Rheum* 8:1145-1151, 1965.(11)

Edathamil in the treatment of scleroderma and calcinosis cutis. (WINDER, P. R. and Curtis, A. C.) *AMA Arch Derm* 82:732-736, 1960. (15)

An objective evaluation of the treatment of systemic scleroderma with disodium EDTA, pyridoxine and reserpine. (FULEIHAN, F. J. D., Kurban, A. K., Abboud, R. T., Beidas-Jubran, N. and Farah, F. S.) *Brit J Derm* 80:184-189, 1968. (20)

Scleroderma. An evaluation of treatment with disodium edetate. (NELDNER, K. H., Winkelmann, R. K. and Perry, H. O.) *Arch Derm* 86:305-309, 1962. (14)

Favorable response of calcinosis universalis to edathamil disodium. (DAVIS, H. and Moe, P. J.) *Pediatrics* 24:780-785, 1959. (18)

Symposium on scleroderma. (Medical Grand Rounds from the University of Alabama Medical Center). (UNIVERSITY OF ALABAMA MEDICAL CENTER. C. Owen, Jr., W. H. Dodson and W. J. Hammack, Editors) *South Med J* 59:1320-1326, 1966. (15)

The treatment of systemic sclerosis with disodium EDTA, pyridoxine and reserpine. (BIRK, R. E. and Rupe, C. E.) *Henry Ford Hosp Med Bull* 14:109-118, 1966. (10)

Systemic sclerosis. Fourteen cases treated with chelation (disodium EDTA) and/or pyridoxine, with comments on the possible role of altered tryptophan metabolism in pathogenesis. (BIRK, R. E. and Rupe, C. E.) *Henry Ford Hosp Med Bull* 10:523-553, 1962. (54)

Therapy of scleroderma with the disodium salt of ethylene diamine tetraacetic acid; a contribution to the toxicology of versenate. Part I. (HOSLI, P.) *Arzneimittelforschung* 10:65-74, 1960. (0)

Diabetes

Chelation therapy of occlusive arteriosclerosis in diabetic patients. (LAMAR, C. P.) *Angiology* 15:379-395, 1964. (33)

Hypoglycaemia induced by disodium ethylene diamine tetraacetic acid. (MELTZER, L. E., Palmon, Jr., F. P. and Kitchell, J. R.) *Lancet* 2:637-638, 1961. (4)

Some physical-chemical variables affecting insulin migration in vitro. I. Electrophoresis. (FREEDLENDER, A. E., Rees, S. B. and Soeldner, J. S.) *Proc Soc Exp Biol Med* 115:21-25, 1964. (7)

EDTA

Spectrophotometric determination of microgram quantities of (ethylenedinitrilo) tetraacetic acid with bis (2, 4, 6-tripyridyl-s-triazine) iron(II). (KRATOCHVIL, B. and White, M. C.) *Anal Chem* 37:111-113, 1965. (14)

Separation of NTA and EDTA chelates by thin-layer chromatography. (RAJABALEE, F. J. M., Potvin, M. and Laham, S.) *J Chromatogr* 79:375-379, 1973. (10)

Infrared spectra and correlations for the ethylene diamine tetraacetic acid metal chelates. (SAWYER, D. T.) *Ann NY Acad Sci* 88:307-321, 1960. (24)

Separation of metal-EDTA complexes by thin-layer chromatography. (VANDER-DEELEN, J.) *J Chromatogr* 39:521-522, 1969. (5)

Ion-exchange characteristics of the radium-ethylene diamine tetraacetate complex. (BAETSLE, L. and Bengsch, E.) *J Chromatogr* 8:265-273, 1962. (10)

Effect of buffer equilibrium on paper electrophoresis. (KABARA, J. J., Zyskowski, D. and Spafford, N.) *J Chromatogr* 13:556-557, 1964. (4)

Coordination chain reactions. II. The ligand-exchange reaction of tetraethylenepentamine-nickel(II) and ethylene diamine tetraacetatocuprate(II). (MARGERUM, D. W. and Carr, J. D.) *J Am Chem Soc* 88:1639-1644, 1966. (13)

Coordination chain reactions. III. The exchange of N, N, N^1, N^1-tetrakis (2-aminoethyl) ethylene diaminezinc(II) and ethylene diamine tetraacetocuprate(II). (CARR, J. D. and Margerum, D. W.) *J Am Chem Soc* 88:1645-1648, 1966. (9)

Alkali metal binding by ethylene diamine tetraacetate, adenosine 5'-triphosphate, and pyrophosphate. (BOTTS, J., Chashin, A. and Young, H. L.) *Biochemistry* 4:1788-1798, 1965. (9)

Base-catalyzed hydrogen-deuterium exchange in bivalent metal-EDTA chelates. (TERRILL, J. B. and Reilley, C. N.) *Anal Chem* 38:1876-1881, 1966. (32)

Anomalous behaviour of EDTA during gel filtration. Studies on the possible contamination of the S100 protein. (LEVI, A., Mercanti, D., Calissano, P. and Alema, S.) *Anal Biochem* 62:301-304, 1974. (6)

EDTA prevents the photocatalyzed destruction of the products of catecholamine oxidation. (KARASAWA, T., Funakoshi, H., Jurukawa, K. and Yoshida, K.) *Anal Biochem* 53:278-281, 1973. (11)

Computation of metal binding in bi-metal — bi-chelate systems. (BOTTS, J., Chashin, A. and Schmidt, L.) *Biochemistry* 5:1360-1364, 1966. (5)

Binding of EDTA to DEAE-cellulose and its interference with protein determinations. (WARD, W. W. and Fastiggi, R. J.) *Anal Biochem* 50:154-162, 1972. (15)

Interference of sodium ethylene diamine tetraacetate in the determination of proteins and its elimination. (NEURATH, A. R.) *Experientia* 22:290, 1966. (2)

Formation constants of certain zinc-complexes by ion-exchange method. (VOHRA, P., Krantz, E. and Kratzer, F. H.) *Proc Soc Exp Biol Med* 121:422-425, 1966. (7)

Gastrointestinal System

Intestines (Human & Animal)
Effects of ethylene diamine tetraacetate and metal ions in intestinal absorption of vitamin B12 in man and rats. (OKUDA, K. and Sasayama, K.) *Proc Soc Exp Biol Med* 120:17-20, 1965. (12)

Intestines (Human)
The action of EDTA on human alkaline phosphatases. (CONYERS, R. A. J., Birkett, D. J., Neale, F. C., Posen, S. and Brudenell-Woods, J.) *Biochim Biophys Acta* 139:363-371, 1967. (44)

Liver (Animal)
The dissociation of rat liver ribosomes by ethylene diamine tetraacetic acid; molecular weights, chemical composition, and buoyant densities of the subunits. (HAMILTON, M. G. and Ruth, M. E.) *Biochemistry* 8:851-856, 1969. (29)

Analytical study of rat liver microsomes treated by EDTA or pyrophosphate. (AMARCOSTESEC, A.) *Arch Int Physiol Biochem* 81:358-359, 1973. (4)

Effect of metal ions and EDTA on the activity of rabbit liver fructose 1,6-diphosphatase. (TATE, S. S.) *Biochem Biophys Res Commun* 24:662-667, 1966. (6)

Liver (Human)
Hepato-lenticular degeneration (Wilson's disease) treated by penicillamine. (RICHMOND, J., Rosenoer, V. M., Tompsett, S. L., Draper, I. and Simpsons, J. A.) *Brain* 87:619-638, 1964. (42)

Hepatolenticular degeneration. Clinical, biochemical and pathologic study of a patient with fulminant course aggravated by treatment with BAL and versenate. (HOLLISTER, L. E., Cull, V. L., Gonda, V. A. and Kolb, F. O.) *Am J Med 28*:623-630, 1960. (16)

Hepatic and renal studies with iron-59 EDTA in patients with and without liver or kidney disease. (McLAREN, J. R., Galambos, J. T. and Drew, W. D.) *Radiology 81*:447-454, 1963. (7)

Genitourinary System

Kidneys (Human)
The effect of glucose on the glomerular filtration rate in normal man. A preliminary report. (BROCHNER-MORTENSEN, J.) *Acta Med Scand 180*:109-111, 1971. (8)

^{51}Cr-EDTA biological half life as an index of renal function. (Letters) (BRIEN, T. G. and Fay, J. A.) *J Nucl Med 13*:339-340, 1972. (4)

Glomerular filtration rate measurement in man by the single injection method using ^{51}Cr-EDTA. (CHANTLER, C., Garnett, E. S., Parsons, V. and Veall, N.) *Clin Sci 37*:169-180, 1969. (27)

^{51}Cr-edetic-acid clearance and G. F. R. (Letters) (STAMP, T. C. B.) *Lancet 2*:1348, 1968. (4)

Comparison between inulin and ^{51}Cr-labelled edetic acid for the measurement of glomerular filtration-rate. (HEATH, D. A., Knapp, M. S. and Walker, W. H. C.) *Lancet 2*:1110-1112, 1968. (18)

Comparison of glomerular filtration rate measurements using inulin, ^{51}Cr-EDTA, and a phosphate infusion technique. (STAMP, T. C. B., Stacey, T. C. and Rose, G. A.) *Clin Chim Acta 30*:351-358, 1970. (20)

A comparison between the clearances of inulin, endogenous creatinine and ^{51}Cr-EDTA. (TRAUB, Y. M., Samuel, R., Lubin, E., Lewitus, Z. and Rosenfeld, J. B.) *Isr J Med Sci 9*:487-489, 1973. (11)

Simultaneous ^{51}Cr edetic acid, inulin, and endogenous creatinine clearances in 20 patients with renal disease. (FAVRE, H. R. and Wing, A. J.) *Brit Med J 1*:84-86, 1968. (11)

Estimation of glomerular filtration rate from plasma clearance of 51-chromium edetic acid. (CHANTLER, C. and Barratt, T. M.) *Arch Dis Child 47*:613-617, 1972. (17)

Dialysance of molecules of different size in reused Kiil, Ab-Gambro, and Rhone-Poulence dialysers. (KRAMER, P., Matthaei, D., Go, J. G., Tonnis, H. J. and Scheler, F.) *Brit Med J 2*:320-322, 1972. (13)

Chemotherapy in nephrolithiasis. (TIMMERMANN, A. and Kallistratos, G.) *Isr J Med Sci 7*:689-695, 1971. (4)

Instrumental chemolysis of renal calculi: indications and dangers. (MISCHOL, H. R. and Wildbolz, R.) *J Urol 105*:607-610, 1971. (21)

Modern aspects of chemical dissolution of human renal calculi by irrigation. (TIMMERMANN, A. and Kallistratos, G.) *J Urol 95*:469-475, 1966. (13)

Uterus (Human)
Effect of EDTA on human cumulus granulosa cells. (DEKEL, N., Shahar, A., Soferman, N. and Kraicer, P. F.) *Isr J Med Sci 8*:2004-2007, 1972. (4)

Immunology

Human Studies

Role of calcium in complement dependent hemolysis. (YACHNIN, S. and Ruthenberg, J.) *Proc Soc Exp Biol Med 117*:179-181, 1964. (12)

Studies on human C'l-esterase. I. Purification and enzymatic properties. (HAINES, A. L. and Lepow, I. H.) *J Immun 92*:456-467, 1964. (25)

Further studies on the effect of Ca + + on the first complement of human complement (C'l). (YOUNG, F. E. and Lepow, I. H.) *J Immun 83*:364-371, 1959. (11)

Lupus Erythematosus

Inhibition of L. E. phenomenon by EDTA. (SAUMUR, J.) *J-Lancet 82*:240-242, 1962. (9)

Methods for the estimation of the second component and third component complex of complement using intermediates of the complement sequence. (TOWNES, A. S. and Stewart, Jr., C. R.) *Bull Hopkins Hosp 117*:331-347, 1965. (17)

Laboratory

Insulin Assay

The immunoassay of insulin in human serum treated with sodium ethylene diamine tetraacetate. (SHELDON, J. and Taylor, K. W.) *J Endocr 33*:157-158, 1965. (5)

Observations on the precipitation reaction in a double-antibody immunoassay for insulin. (GRANT, D. B.) *Acta Endocr 59*:139-149, 1968. (10)

Influence of heparin-plasma, EDTA-plasma, and serum on the determination of insulin with three different radioimmunoassays. (THORELL, J. I. and Lanner, A.) *Scand J Clin Lab Invest 31*:187-190, 1973. (15)

Urinalysis

Transport of urine specimens for bacteriological examination. Experiment with addition of calcium disodium edathamil. (ODEGAARD, K. and Odegaard, A.) *Nord Med 81*:607-609, 1969. (14)

Chelatometric magnesium determination in urine. (WUNSCH, L.) *Clin Chim Acta 30*:157-163, 1970. (10)

Quantitative determination of EDTA and other polyamino acetic acids in urine and serum. (STAHLAVSKA, A. and Malat, M.) *Clin Chim Acta 41*:181-186, 1972. (19)

Spectrophotometric determination of ethylene diamine tetraacetic acid in plasma and urine. (LAVENDER, A. R., Pullman, T. N. and Goldman, D.) *J Lab Clin Med 63*:299-305, 1964. (8)

A simple method for the determination of EDTA in serum and urine. (BLIJENBERG, B. G. and Leijnse, B.) *Clin Chim Acta 26*:577-579, 1969. (1)

Simple and precise micromethod for EDTA titration of calcium. (COPP, D. H., Cheney, G. A. and Stokoe, N. M.) *J Lab Clin Med 61*:1029-1037, 1963. (11)

Determination of calcium in urine with EDTA by means of a cation exchange resin. (VEDSO, S. and Rud, C.) *Scand J Clin Lab Invest 15*:395-398, 1963. (6)

Potentiometric determinations of calcium, magnesium, and complexing agents in water and biological fluids. (RIET, B. VAN'T and Wynn. J. E.) *Anal Chem* 41:158-162, 1969. (3)

Lipids

Human Studies
A procedure for in vitro studies on fatty acid metabolism by human subcutaneous adipose tissue. (OSTMAN, J.) *Acta Med Scand* 177:183-197, 1965.

Microbiology

Enzymes (Lysozyme)
Effects of organic cations on the gram-negative cell wall and their bactericidal activity with ethylene diamine tetraacetate and surface active agents. (VOSS, J. G.) *J Gen Microbiol* 48:391-400, 1967. (21)

Effect of ethylene diamine tetraacetic acid, Triton X-100, and lysozyme on the morphology and chemical composition of/isolated cell walls of *Escherichia coli*. (SCHNAITMAN, C. A.) *J Bact* 108:553-563, 1971. (20)

Lysis of *Escherichia coli* with a neutral detergent. (GODSON, G. N. and Sinsheimer, R. L.) *Biochim Biophys Acta* 149:476-488, 1967. (16)

The role of amine buffers in EDTA toxicity and their effect on osmotic shock. (NEU, H. C.) *J Gen Microbiol* 57:215-220, 1969. (11)

Sensitization of *E. coli* to the serum bactericidal system and to lysozyme by ethyleneglycol-tetraacetic acid. (BRYAN, C. S.) *Proc Soc Exp Biol Med* 145:1431-1433, 1974. (8)

Musculoskeletal System

Muscles (Human)
Reversal of the ATPase reaction in muscle fibres by EDTA. (DREWS, G. A. and Engel, W. K.) *Nature* 212:1551-1553, 1966. (24)

Myositis ossificans traumatica with unusual course. Effect of EDTA on calcium, phosphorus and manganese excretion. (LIBERMAN, U. A., Barzel, U., De Vries, A. and Ellis, H.) *Am J Med Sci* 254:35-47, 1967. (50)

Capillary permeability to human skeletal muscle measured by local injection of ^{51}Cr-EDTA and ^{133}Xe. (TRAP-JENSEN, J., Korsgaard, O. and Lassen, N. A.) *Scand J Clin Lab Invest* 25:93-99, 1970. (23)

Tendons (Human)
An electron microscopic study of the effect of crude bacterial a-amylase and ethylene diamine tetraacetic acid on human tendon. (DIXON, J. S., Hunter, J. A. A. and Steven, F. S.) *J Ultrastruct Red* 38:466-472, 1972. (12)

Neuropsychiatric

Human Studies

ACTH and a chelating agent for schizophrenia. (KEBE, S. R.) *West Med* 4:46, 48, 1963. (6)

Porphyric psychosis and chelation therapy. (PETERS, H. A.) *Recent Adv Biol Psychiat* 4:204-217, 1961. (31)

Abnormal copper and tryptophan metabolism and chelation therapy in anticonvulsant drug intolerance. (PETERS, H. A., Eichman, P. L., Price, J. M., Kozelka, F. L. and Reese, H. H.) *Dis Nerv Syst* 27:97-107, 1966. (26)

Pyruvic and lactic acid metabolism in muscular dystrophy, neuropathies and other neuromuscular disorders. (GOTO, I., Peters, H. A. and Reese, H. H.) *Am J Med Sci* 253:431-448, 1967. (24)

Nucleic Acids

Animal Studies

The release of radioactive nucleic acids and mucoproteins by trypsin and ethylene diamine tetraacetate treatment of baby-hamster cells in tissue culture. (SNOW, C. and Allen A.) *Biochem J* 119:707-714, 1970. (31)

Structural studies on ribosomes. II. Denaturation and sedimentation of ribosomal subunits unfolded in EDTA. (MIALL, S. H. and Walker, I. O.) *Biochem Biophys Acta* 174:551-560, 1969. (15)

The dissociation of rabbit reticulocyte ribosomes with EDTA and the location of messenger ribonucleic acid. (NOLAN, R. D. and Arnstein, H. R. V.) *Europ J Biochem* 9:445-450, 1969. (22)

Evidence for the detachment of a ribonucleoprotein messenger complex from EDTA-treated rabbit reticulocyte polyribosomes. (TEMMERMAN, J. and Lebleu, B.) *Biochim Biophys Acta* 174:544-550, 1969. (11)

The degradation of deoxyribonucleic acid by L-cysteine and the promoting effect of metal chelating agents and of catalase. (BERNEIS, K. and Kofler, M.) *Experientia* 20:16-17, 1964. (13)

A differential solvent effect on thermal stability of genetic markers in DNA. (PETERSON, J. M. and Guild, W. R.) *J Mol Biol* 20:497-503, 1966. (16)

The influence of chelating agents on the prooxidative effect of a hydrogen peroxide producing methylhydrazine compound. (BERNEIS, K., Kofler, M. and Bollag, W.) *Experientia* 20:73-74, 1964. (9)

Nucleotides and Nucleosides

Animal Studies

Studies of the 105,000 X g supernatant of different rat tissues. (MORGAN, W. S.) *Lab Invest* 12:968-977, 1963. (10)

Coelomocyte aggregation in *Cucumaria frondosa*: effect of ethylene diamine tetraacetate, adenosine, and adenosine nucleotides. (NOBLE, P. B.) *Biol Bull* 139:549-556, 1970. (17)

Nutrition

Animal Studies
Calcium utilization and feed efficiency in the growing rat as affected by dietary calcium, buffering capacity, lactose and EDTA. (EVANS, J. L. and Ali, R.) *J Nutr* 92:417-424, 1967. (36)

Effects of dietary EDTA and cadmium on absorption, excretion and retention of orally administered ^{65}Zn in various tissues of zinc-deficient and normal goats and calves. (POWELL, G. W., Miller, W. J. and Blackmon, D. M.) *J Nutr* 93:203-212, 1967. (34)

Quantitative relation of EDTA to availability of zinc for turkey poults. (KRATZER, F. H. and Starcher, B.) *Proc Soc Exp Biol Med* 113:424-426, 1963. (3)

Metabolism of ethylene diamine tetraacetic acid (EDTA) by chickens. (DARWISH, N. M. and Kratzer, F. H.) *J Nutr* 86:187-192, 1965. (16)

Effects of the apical ectodermal ridge on growth of the Versene-stripped chick limb bud. (GASSELING, M. T. and Saunders, Jr., J. W.) *Develop Biol* 3:1-25, 1961. (35)

Iron Metabolism (Animal)
A study of the prolonged intake of small amounts of ethylene diamine tetraacetate on the utilization of low dietary levels of calcium and iron by the rat. (HAWKINS, W. W., Leonard, V. G., Maxwell, J. E. and Rastogi, K. S.) *Canad J Biochem* 40:391-395, 1962. (5)

The effect of ingestion of disodium ethylene diamine tetraacetate on the absorption and metabolism of radioactive iron by the rat. (LARSEN, B. A., Bidwell, R. G. and Hawkins, W. W.) *Canad J Biochem* 38:51-55, 1960. (11)

The effect of prolonged intake of ethylene diamine tetraacetate on the utilization of calcium and iron by the rat. (LARSEN, B. A., Hawkins, W. W., Leonard, V. G. and Armstrong, J. E.) *Canad J Biochem* 38:813-817, 1960. (7)

Fe^{59}-amino acid complexes: are they intermediates in Fe^{59} absorption across intestinal mucosa? (MANIS, J. and Schachter, D.) *Proc Soc Exp Biol Med* 119:1185-1187, 1965. (5)

Iron Metabolism (Human)
Clinical usefulness of iron chelating agents. (WAXMAN, H. S. and Brown, E. B.) *Progr Hematol* 6:338-373, 1969. (138)

A comparative study of iron absorption and utilization following ferrous suphate and sodium ironedetate ("Sytron®"). (HODGKINSON, R.) *Med J Aust* 1:809-811, 1961. (6)

Factors influencing the clinical use of chelates in iron storage disease. (WEINER, M.) *Ann NY Acad Sci* 119:789-796, 1964. (27)

Effect of orally administered chelating agents EDTA, DTPA and fructose on radioiron absorption in man. (DAVIS, P. S. and Deller, D. J.) *Aust Ann Med* 16:70-74, 1967. (15)

Life Extension (Animal)
Life extension in the rotifer *Mytilina brevispina var redunca* by the application of chelating agents. (SINCOCK, A. M.) *J Geront* 30:289-293, 1975. (5)

Zinc Metabolism (Human)
Fate of intravenously administered zinc chelates in man. (ROSOFF, B., Hart, H., Methfessel, A. H. and Spencer, H.) *J Appl Physiol 30*:12-16, 1971. (30)

Ophthalmology

Human Studies
Scleromalacia perforans associated with Crohn's disease treated with sodium versenate (EDTA). (EVANS, P. J. and Eustace, P.) *Brit J Ophthal 57*:330-335, 1973. (12)

Effect of intravenous sodium bicarbonate, disodium edetate (Na_2EDTA), and hyperventilation on visual and oculomotor signs in multiple sclerosis. (DAVIS, F. A., Becker, F. O., Michael, J. A. and Sorensen, E.) *J Neurol Neurosurg Psychiat 33*:723-732, 1970. (34)

Treatment of blepharitis. (BARAS, I.) *Eye Ear Nose Throat Mon 44*:68, 70, 118, Feb. 1965. (10)

Corneal contact lens solutions. (GOULD, H. L. and Inglima, R.) *Eye Ear Nose Throat Mon 43*:39-49, Apr. 1964. (8)

A new technique of contact lens storage, soaking and cleaning. (DABEZIES, JR., O. H. and Naugle, T.) *Eye Ear Nose Throat Mon 50*:378-382, Oct. 1971. (3)

Otolaryngology

Animal Studies
Biological study of a chelating agent with an affinity for calcium in the field of otology. (CHEVANCE, L. G.) *Acta Otolaryng 51*:46-54, 1960. (0)

Human Studies
Chelation therapy in Wegener's granulomatosis. Treatment with EDTA. (HANSOTIA, P., Peters, H., Bennett, M. and Brown, R.) *Ann Otol 78*:388-402, 1969. (27)

Chelation in clinical otosclerosis. (STECKER, R. H. and Bennett, M.) *AMA Arch Otolaryng 70*:627-629, 1959. (8)

Poisoning

Chelation in medicine. (SCHUBERT, J.) *Sci Am 214*:40-50, 1966. (0)

Chelation. (RENOUX, M. and Mikol, C.) *Presse Med 72*:3317-3319, 1964. (0)

Clinical uses of metal-binding drugs. (CHENOWORTH, M. B.) *Clin Pharmacol Ther 9*:365-387, 1968. (251)

Lead (Alcohol)
Clinical manifestations and therapy of acute lead intoxication due to the ingestion of illicitly distilled alcohol. (CRUTCHER, J. C.) *Ann Intern Med 59*:707-715, 1963. (22)

Lead intoxication and alcoholism: a diagnostic dilemma. (CRUTCHER, J. C.) *J Med Assoc Georgia 56*:1-4, Jan. 1967. (15)

Chelation therapy in lead nephropathy. (MORGAN, J. M.) *South Med J 68*:1001-1006, 1975. (18)

Treatment of lead intoxication. Combined use of peritoneal dialysis and edetate calcium disodium. (MEHBOD, H.) *JAMA 201*:972-974, 1967. (4)

Porphyrin metabolism during Versenate® therapy in lead poisoning. Intoxication from an unusual source. (FROMKE, V. L., Lee, M. Y. and Watson, C. J.) *Ann Intern Med 70*:1007-1012, 1969. (29)

Lead (Children)

Treatment of lead encephalopathy. The combined use of edetate and hemodialysis. (SMITH, H. D., King, L. R. and Margolin, E. G.) *Am J Dis Child 109*:322-324, 1965. (6)

Erythrocyte hypoplasia due to lead poisoning. A devastating, yet curable disease. (MOOSA, A. and Harris, F.) *Clin Pediat 8*:404-402, 1969. (13)

Successful calcium disodium ethylene diamine tetraacetate treatment of lead poisoning in an infant. (KNELLER, L. A., Uhl, H. S. M. and Brem, Jr.) *New Eng J Med 252*:338-340, 1955. (16)

Lead intoxication in children: a current problem in Providence, Rhode Island. Appearance of 19 cases of lead poisoning in children in two year period constitutes epidemic. (ORSON, J. and May, J. B.) *Rhode Island Med J 48*:608-611, 1965. (3)

Ambulatory treatment of lead poisoning: report of 1,155 cases. (SACHS, H. K., Blanksma, L. A., Murray, E. F. and O'Connell, M. J.) *Pediatrics 46*:389-396, 1970. (5)

Lead poisoning from home remedies. (McNEIL, J. R. and Reinhard, M. C.) *Clin Pediat 6*:150-156, 1967. (25)

Lead neuropathy in children. (SETO, D. S. Y. and Freeman, J. M.) *Am J Dis Child 107*:337-342, 1964. (21)

The use of chelating agents in the treatment of acute and chronic lead intoxication in childhood. (CHISOLM, JR., J. J.) *J Pediat 73*:1-38, 1968. (92)

Treatment of lead encephalopathy in children. (COFFIN, R., Phillips, J. L., Staples, W. I. and Spector, S) *J Pediat 69*:198-206, 1966. (28)

Reversible myocarditis due to chronic lead poisoning in childhood. (FREEMAN, R.) *Arch Dis Child 40*:389-393, 1965. (23)

Lead poisoning. (Accidental chemical poisonings.) (JACOBZINER, H. and Raybin, H. W.) *New York J Med 63*:2999-3001, 1963. (0)

Treatment of lead poisoning with intramuscular edathamil calcium-disodium. (SHRAND, H.) *Lancet 1*:310-312, 1961. (25)

Chelation therapy in children with subclinical plumbish. (CHISOLM, JR., J. J.) *Pediatrics 53*:441-443, 1974. (17)

Lead poisoning in children. (Clinical Rounds from the Massachusetts General Hospital). (FEIGIN, R. D., Shannon, D. C., Reynolds, S. L., Shapiro, L. W. and Connelly, J. P.) *Clin Pediat 4*:38-45, 1965. (13)

Calcium disodium edathamil therapy of lead intoxication. The significance of aminoaciduria. (ANDREWS, B. F.) *Arch Environ Health 3*:563-567, 1961. (27)

Lead poisoning in children. (MONCRIEFF, A. A., Koumides, O. P., Clayton, B. E., Patrick, A. D., Renwick, A. G. C. and Roberts, G. E.) *Arch Dis Child 39*:1-13, 1964. (29)

Lead (Pregnancy)
Lead poisoning during pregnancy. Fetal tolerance of calcium disodium edetate. (ANGLE, C. R. and McIntire, M. S.) *Am J Dis Child 108*:436-439, 1964.

Mercury
The treatment of chronic intoxications due to lead, arsenic and mercury. (LEWIS, C. E.) *GP 27*:128-132, 1963. (0)

Acrodynia. A long-term study of 62 cases. (CHAMBERLAIN, 3rd, J. L. and Quillian, II, W. W.) *Clin Pediat 2*:439-443, 1963. (16)

A controlled trial of edathamil calcium disodium in acrodynia. (McCOY, J. E., Carre, I. J. and Freeman, M.) *Pediatrics 25*:304-308, 1960. (24)

Plutonium (Human)
Plutonium excretion. Study following treatment with zirconium citrate and edathamil calcium-disodium. (SANDERS, JR., S. M.) *Arch Environ Health 2*:474-483, 1961. (27)

Selenium (Animal)
The treatment of acute selenium, cadmium, and tungsten intoxication in rats with calcium disodium ethylene diamine tetraacetate. (SIVJAKOV, K. I. and Braun, H. A.) *Toxicol Appl Pharmacol 1*:602-608, 1959. (15)

Snakes
The chemical modification of necrogenic and proteolytic activities of venom and the use of EDTA to produce *Agkistrodon piscivorus*, a venom toxoid. (GOUCHER, C. R. and Flowers, H. H.) *Toxicon 2*:139-147, 1964. (10)

The effect of EDTA on the extent of tissue damage caused by the venoms of *Bothrops atrox* and *Agkistrodon piscivorus*. (FLOWERS, H. H. and Goucher, C. R.) *Toxicon 2*:221-224, 1965. (7)

Studies on the improvement of treatment of Habu snake (*Trimeresurus flavoviridis*) bite. 2. Antitoxic action of monocalcium disodium ethylene diamine tetraacetate on Habu venom. (SAWAI, Y., Makino, M., Miyasaki, S., Kawamura, Y., Mitsuhashi, S. and Okonogi, T.) *Jap J Exp Med 31*:267-275, 1961. (8)

Radiology

Promotion of radioisotope excretion. (STRAIN, W. H., Danahy, D. T., O'Reilly, R. J., Thomas, M. R., Wilson, R. M. and Pories, W. J.) *J Nucl Med 8*:110-116, 1967. (7)

Effect of multiple injections of calcium compounds on the survival of x-irradiated rats. (RIXON, R. H. and Whitfield, J. R.) *Nature 199*:821-822, 1963. (15)

Distribution of cobalt-60 in the rat as influenced by chelating agents. (DU KHUONG LE) *Nature 204*:696-697, 1964. (10)

Respiratory System

Animal Studies
Intravascular concentrations of calcium and magnesium ions and edema formation in isolated lungs. (NICOLAYSEN, G.) *Acta Physiol Scand 81*:325-339, 1971. (22)

Ultrastructural studies of the alveolar-capillary barrier in isolated plasma-perfused rabbit lungs. Effects of EDTA and of increased capillary pressure. (HOVIG, T., Nicolaysen, A. and Nicolaysen, G.) *Acta Physiol Scand 82*:417-431, 1971. (13)

The importance of decalcification in the treatment of tuberculosis. III. The influence of decalcification of the course of experimental tuberculosis in guinea pigs infected with tubercle bacilli of low degree resistance to izoniazid. (GARAPICH, M., Jelonek, A. and Kulig, A.) *Acta Med Pol 8*:313-318, 1967. (6)

The importance of decalcification in the treatment of tuberculosis. I. The influence of decalcification in the course of healing in experimental tuberculosis in guinea pigs. (GIZA, T., Hanicka, M., Jelonek, A., Kulig, A., Rembiesowa, H. and Garapich, M.) *Acta Paediat Scand 55*:33-37, 1966. (9)

Human Studies
Measurement of sputum viscosity in a cone-plate viscometer. II. An evaluation of mycolytic agents in vitro. (LIEBERMAN, J.) *Am Rev Resp Dis 97*:662-672, 1968. (24)

Rheumatoid Arthritis

Some in vivo effects of chelation. I. Rheumatoid arthritis. (BOYLE, A. J., Mosher, R. E. and McCann, D. S.) *J Chron Dis 16*:325-328, 1963. (5)

Case histories of rheumatoid arthritis treated with sodium or magnesium EDTA. (LEIPZIG, L. J., Boyle, A. J. and McCann, D. S.) *J Chron Dis 22*:553-563, 1970. (22)

Toxicity Studies

Animal Studies
Safety evaluation studies of calcium EDTA. (OSER, B. L., Oser, M. and Spencer, H. C.) *Toxicol Appl Pharmacol 5*:142-162, 1963. (4)

The toxicity and pharmacodynamics of EGTA: oral administration to rats and comparisons with EDTA. (WYNN, J. E., Riet, B. Van't and Borzelleca, J. F..) *Toxicol Appl Pharmacol 16*:807-817, 1970. (6)

The relative toxicity in rats of disodium ethylene diamine tetraacetate, sodium oxalate and sodium citrate. (PAYNE, J. M. and Sansom, B. F.) *J Physiol 170*:613-620, 1964. (2)

Metabolic changes in experimental poisoning with ethylene diamine tetraacetic acid. (REMAGEN, W., Hiller, F. K. and Sanz, C. M.) *Arzneimittelforschung 11*:1097-1099, 1961. (22)

Contribution to the metabolism of $MnNa_2$ edathamil. (SYKORA, J., Kocher, Z. and Eybl, V.) *AMA Arch Indust Health 21*:24-27, 1960. (6)

The toxic effect of $CoCl_2$, Co(Co-EDTA) or Na_2(Co-EDTA) containing aerosols on the rat and the distribution of (Co-EDTA) — in guinea pig organs. (HOBEL, M., Maroske, D., Wegener, K. and Eichler, O.) *Arch Int Pharmacodyn Ther 198*:213-222, 1972. (5)

Human Studies
Chelation therapy. (CRAVEN, P. C. and Morrelli, H. F.) *West J Med 122*:277-278, 1975. (14)

Toxic side effects of ethylene diamine tetraacetic acid. (FOREMAN, H.) *J Chron Dis* 16:319-323, 1963. (20)

The long term use, side effects, and toxicity of disodium ethylene diamine tetraacetic acid (EDTA). (MELTZER, L. E., Kitchell, J. R. and Palmon, Jr., F.) *Am J Med Sci* 242:11-17, 1961. (37)

Acute versenate nephrosis occurring as the result of treatment for lead intoxication. (REUBER, M. D. and Bradley, J. E.) *JAMA 174*:263-269, 1960. (17)

Fatal nephropathy during edathamil therapy in lead poisoning. (BRUGSCH, H. G.) *AMA Arch Indust Health 20*:285-292, 1959. (41)

Pathologic changes associated with the use of sodium ethylene diamine tetraacetate in the treatment of hypercalcemia. (DUDLEY, H. R., Ritchie, A. C., Schilling, A. and Baker, W. H.) *New Eng J Med 252*:331-337, 1955. (43)

Hazards of edathamil (EDTA) therapy in lead intoxication. (Letters) (ANDREWS, B. F.) *Pediatrics 28*:161-162, 1961. (6)

Lesions resembling vitamin B complex deficiency and urinary loss of zinc produced by ethylene diamine tetraacetate. (PERRY, JR., H. M. and Schroeder. H. A.) *Am J Med* 22:168-172, 1957. (11)

Edetic acid therapy. (Letters) (NODINE, J. H.) *JAMA 212*:628, 1970. (6)

Kidneys (Animal)
A comparative study of the toxic effects of calcium and chromium chelates of ethylene diamine tetraacetate in the dog. (AHRENS, F. A. and Aronson, A. L.) *Toxicol Appl Pharmacol 18*:10-25, 1971. (32)

Study of the mechanism of renal vacuologenesis induced in the rat by ethylene diamine tetraacetate. Comparison of the cellular activities of calcium and chromium chelates. (SCHWARTZ, S. L., Johnson, C. B. and Doolan, P. D.) *Mol Pharmacol* 6:54-60, 1970. (11)

Calcium disodium edetate nephrosis in female rats of varying ages. (REUBER, M. D.) *J Path 97*:335-338, 1969. (16)

Subcellular localization of ethylene diamine tetraacetate in the proximal tubular cell of the rat kidney. (SCHWARTZ, S. L., Johnson, C. B., Hayes, J. R. and Doolan, P. D.) *Biochem Pharmacol 16*:2413-2419, 1967. (17)

An evaluation of the nephrotoxicity of ethylene diamine tetraacetate and diethylene triamine pentaacetate in the rat. (DOOLAN, P. D., Schwartz, S. L., Hayes, J. R., Mullen, J. C. and Cummings, N. B.) *Toxicol Appl Pharmacol 10*:481-500, 1967. (36)

Calcium disodium edetate nephrosis in inbred rats. Variation in Marshall, Buffalo, Fisher, and ACI strains. (REUBER, M. D. and Lee, C. W.) *Arch Environ Health 13*:554-557, 1966. (13)

Studies of the nephrotoxicity of ethylene diamine tetraacetic acid. (SCHWARTZ, S. L., Hayes, J. R., Ide, R. S., Johnson, C. B. and Doolan, P. D.) *Biochem Pharmacol* 15:377-389, 1966. (24)

Effects of edathamil disodium on the kidney. (ALTMAN, J., Wakim, K. G. and Winkelmann, R. K.) *J Invest Derm 38*:215-218, 1962. (5)

Edetate kidney lesions in rats. (REUBER, M. D. and Schmieler, G. C.) *Arch Environ Health 5*:430-436, 1962. (23)

Kidneys (Human & Animal)

Nephrotoxic hazard from uncontrolled edathamil calcium-disodium therapy. (FOREMAN, H., Finnegan, C. and Lushbaugh, C. C.) *JAMA 160*:1042-1046, 1956. (7)

Accentuation of Ca edetate nephrosis by cortisone. (REUBER, M. D.) *Arch Path 76*:382-386, 1963. (18)

Liver (Animal)

'Phenergan' and versene in dietary liver necrosis. (McLEAN, A. E. M.) *Nature 185*:191-192, 1960. (4)

Hepatic lesions in young rats given calcium disodium edetate. *Pharmacol 11*:321-326, 1967. (14)

Teratology (Animal)

Chelating agents and teratogenesis. (Letters) (MARSH, L. and Fraser, F. C.) *Lancet 1*:846, 1973. (29)

A direct analysis of early chick embryonic neuroepithelial responses following exposure to EDTA. (DANIELS, E. and Moore, K. L.) *Teratology 6*:215-225, 1972. (25)

Teratogenic effects of a chelating agent and their prevention by zinc. (SWENERTON, H. and Hurley, L. A.) *Science 173*:62-64, 1971. (16)

Tumors and Viruses

Animal Studies

Studies on cell deformability. III. Some effects of EDTA on sarcoma 37 cells. (WEISS, L.) *J Cell Biol 33*:341-347, 1967. (23)

Chelating agents for the binding of metal ions to macromolecules. (SUNDBERG, M. W., Meares, C. F., Goodwin, D. A. and Diamanti, C. L.) *Nature 250*:587-588, 1974. (9)

Inhibition of DNA synthesis in animal cells by ethylene diamine tetraacetate, and its reversal by zinc. (RUBIN, H.) *Proc Natl Acad Sci USA 69*:712-716, 1972. (15)

Some effects of disodium ethylene diamine tetraacetate on the growth of transplantable mouse tumors. (ASANO, M.) *Jap J Med Sci Biol 12*:365-374, 1959. (15)

Local inhibition and enhancement of growth of transplanted tumor cells in mice. (GITLITZ, G. F., Ship, A. G., Glick, J. L. and Glick, A. H.) *J Surg Res 3*:370-376, 1963. (32)

Human Studies

Studies of cell deformability." IV. A possible role of calcium in cell contact phenomena. (WEISS, L.) *J Cell Biol 35*:347-356, 1967. (34)

Metals, ligands, and cancer. (WILLIAMS, D. R.) *Chem Rev 72*:203-213, 1972. (108)

The effect of anticoagulants on the volume of normal and leukemic leukocytes. (LADINSKY, J. L. and Westring, D. W.) *Cancer Res 27*:1689-1695, 1967. (22)

Sustaining Member-Physicians of the Academy

ALABAMA

H. Ray Evers, M.D.
Evers Health Center
Sealy Springs Health Services, Inc.
P.O. Drawer 587
Cottonwood, Alabama 36320

ALASKA

Paul G. Isaak, M.D.
Box 569
Soldotna, Alaska 99669

ARIZONA

Lloyd D. Armold, D.O.
2525 S. Rural Road
Suite 4 North
Tempe, Arizona 85282

Stanley R. Olsztyn, M.D.
3302 N. Miller Road
Scottsdale, Arizona 85251

Robert Wickman, D.O.
1525 N. Granite Reef Road
Scottsdale, Arizona 85257

ARKANSAS

Norbert J. Becquet, M.D., C.M.D.
115 W. 6th
Little Rock, Arkansas

CALIFORNIA

H. Clay Barton, M.D.
1125 E. 17th Street
Suite E.224
Santa Ana, California 92701

H. Richard Casdorph, M.D.
1729 Termino Avenue, Suite A
Long Beach, California 90804

Joseph J. Cyr, M.D.
1920 E. Katella
Orange, California 92667

Orville J. Davis, M.D.
4224 Ohio Street
San Diego, California 92104

Carl Ebnother, M.D.
925 East Meadow
Palo Alto, California 94303

Michael Lee Gerber, M.D.
45 Camino Alto
Mill Valley, California 94941

Robert B. Gold, D.O.
1905 North College Avenue B-2
Santa Ana, California 90270

William J. Goldwag, M.D.
7499 Cerritos Avenue
Stanton, California 90680

Garry F. Gordon, M.D.
8383 Wilshire Blvd.
Suite 922
Beverly Hills, California 90211

Ross Gordon, M.D.
405 Kains Avenue
Albany, California 94706

Bruce Halstead, M.D.
11155 Mt. View Avenue, Suite A
Loma Linda, California 92354

Harold Harper, M.D.
11311 Camarillo St. #103
No. Hollywood, California 91602

Robert Haskell, M.D.
5133 Geary Blvd.
San Francisco, California 94118

James J. Julian, M.D.
1654 Cahuenga at Hollywood Blvd.
Hollywood, California 90028

Richard D. Kaplan, D.O.
3382 Sacramento Street
San Francisco, California 94118

A. Leonard Klepp, M.D.
16311 Ventura Blvd.
Suite 725
Encino, California 91436

Michael Kwiker, D.O.
2811 "L" Street
Sacramento, California 95821

Carl V. Lansing, M.D.
1200 Marshall Street
Crescent City, California 95531

Peter V. Madill, M.D.
6875 Walker Avenue
Sebastopol, California 95472

Donald E. Medaris, M.D.
638 W. Duarte Road
Suite 8
Arcadia, California 91006

Carrol C. Mendenhall, M.D.
255 Crestview Drive
Santa Clara, California 95050

Antonio E.J. Monti, M.D.
505 No. Mollison Avenue
El Cajon, California 92021

Frank J. Mosler, M.D.
14428 Gilmore Street
Van Nuys, California 91401

Luigi Pacini, M.D.
1307 N. Commerce
Stockton, California 95202

William J. Saccoman, M.D.
505 No. Mollison Avenue
El Cajon, California 92021

David A. Steenblock, D.O.
22821 Lake Forest Drive, #112
El Toro, California 92630

Murray R. Susser, M.D.
6552 Bolsa Avenue
Huntington Beach, California 92647

Elmer Thomassen, M.D.
408 Westminister Avenue
Newport Beach, California 92660

Mortimer Weiss, M.D.
1580 E. Washington
Petaluma, California 94952

COLORADO

John F. Bumpus, D.O.
Suite 350
Cherry Terrace Med. Bldg.
3865 Cherry Creek North Drive
Denver, Colorado 80209

William Doell, D.O.
5715 Wadsworth Bypass
Aurora, Colorado 80002

FLORIDA

Douglas M. Baird, D.O.
630 U.S. One
North Palm Beach, Florida 33458

Donald J. Carrow, M.D.
147 N. Belcher Road, Suite 4
Largo, Florida 33541

Daniel G. Clark, M.D.
67 W. Granada Avenue
Ormond Beach, Florida 32074

Charles E. Curtis, D.O.
310 U.S. Highway #1
Lake Park, Florida 33403

Joseph DiStefano, Ph.D.
1481 Belleair Road
Clearwater, Florida 33516

George F. Graves, Jr. D.O.
1481 Belleair Road
Clearwater, Florida 33516

E. Randall Horton, D.O.
3202—42nd Street
West Bradenton, Florida 33505

Clarence W. Lynn, M.D.
1900 N. Orange Avenue
Orlando, Florida 32804

Alfred S. Massam, M.D.
P.O. Box 1328
Wauchula, Florida 33873

Wilfred W. Mittelstadt, D.O.
4747 N. Ocean Blvd.
Suite 200
Ft. Lauderdale, Florida 33308

Robert G. Panzer, D.O.
3005 S.W. 70th. Lane
Gainesville, Florida 32601

Walter C. Parsons, D.O.
4700—9th Avenue North
St. Petersburg, Florida 33713

Robert J. Rogers, M.D.
15 W. Avenue B
Melbourne, Florida 32901

Ricardo J. Sabates, M.D.
1421 E. Oakland Park Blvd.
Ft. Lauderdale, Florida 33319

Lester I. Tavel, D.O., M.D.
401 Manatee Avenue E.
Bradenton, Florida 33508

Watson A. Walden, N.D.
P.O. Drawer WW—2101 McGregor Blvd.
Ft. Myers, Florida 33902

GEORGIA

William C. Douglass, M.D.
41 Perimeter Way, N.W.
Atlanta, Georgia

HAWAII

James E. Baum, D.O.
2158 Main Street, #103-105
Wailuku, Hawaii 96793

Richard Renn, D.O.
Hilton Hawaiian Village
Honolulu, Hawaii 96815

ILLINOIS

M. Paul Dommers, M.D.
303 Andrews Drive
Belvidere, Illinois 61008

Robert Helms, Jr. M.B.A., C.P.A.
American International Hospital
Shiloh Blvd.
Zion, Illinois 60099

William J. Mauer, D.O.
1819—27th Street
Zion, Illinois 60099

Ralph H. Roeper, D.O.
121 N. Northwest Highway
Palatine, Illinois 60067

Ranulfo Sanchez, M.D.
1911 27th Street
Zion, Illinois 60999

John R. Tambone, M.D.
102 E. South Street
Woodstock, Illinois 60098

INDIANA

Floyd B. Coleman, M.D.
405 S. Wayne
Waterloo, Indiana 46793

Martin Lushbough, D.O.
100 South Main Street
North Liberty, Indiana 46554

Harold Sparks, D.O.
3001 Washington Avenue
Evansville, Indiana 47714

Wilbert Streeter, D.O.
3313—45th.
Highland, Indiana 46322

David E. Turfler, D.O.
336 W. Navarre Street
So. Bend, Indiana 46616

KANSAS

Stevens B. Acker, M.D.
3126 E. Central
Wichita, Kansas 67214

Terry R. Hunsberger, D.O.
602 N. Third, P.O. Box 679
Garden City, Kansas 67846

Alfred H. Thiemann, D.O.
301 Derby
Sublette, Kansas 67877

MARYLAND

Hellfried E. Sartori, M.D.
4808 Macon Road
Rockville, Maryland 20852

MICHIGAN

Vahagn Agbabian, D.O.
1105 Pontiac State Bank Bldg.
28 North Saginaw Street
Pontiac, Michigan 48058

Norman E. Clark, M.D.
21950 Greenfield Road
Oak Park, Michigan 48237

Adam Frent, D.O.
33611 Warren Road
Westland, Michigan 48185

Ole C. Kistler, D.O.
12100 Dix—Toledo Road
Southgate, Michigan 48195

Michael T. Nadolny, D.O.
8623 N. Wayne Road, #357
Westland, Michigan 48185

Albert J. Scarchilli, D.O.
Farmington Hills Center for
Preventive Medicine
30275 Thirteen Mile Road
Farmington Hills, Michigan 40818

Richard E. Tapert, D.O.
15850 E. Warren Avenue
Detroit, Michigan 48224

MISSOURI

W.W. Brentlinger, D.O.
2800 A. Kendallwood Parkway
Gladstone, Missouri 64119

Edward McDonagh, D.O.
2800 A. Kendallwood Parkway
Gladstone, Missouri 64119

Albert Leo Pfauth, D.O.
102 Collette Street
Excelsior Springs, Missouri 64024

Charles J. Rudolph, D.O., Ph.D.
2800 A Kendallwood Parkway
Kansas City, Missouri 64119

James E. Swann, D.O.
2425 S. Crysler
Independence, Missouri 64052

Harvey Walker, Jr. M.D., Ph.D.
138 North Meramec Avenue
Clayton, Missouri 63105

NEVADA

Yiwen Y. Tang, M.D.
290 Brinkly Road
Reno, Nevada 89509

NEW MEXICO

Paul V. Wynn, D.O.
4123 Montgomery Blvd.
Albuquerque, New Mexico 87109

NEW JERSEY

John L. Klauber, M.D.
70 Rock Road
Englewood Cliffs, New Jersey 07632

NEW YORK

Warren M. Levin, M.D.
#5 World Trade Center #367
New York City, N.Y. 10048

Harold Markus, M.D.
30 E. 60th Street, Suite 1108
New York, N.Y. 10022

Michael B. Schachter, M.D.
Mountainview Medical Bldg.
Mountainview Avenue
Nyack, New York 10960

I. Sanford Schwartz, R.D.N.D.
New York Center for Holistic
Health & Sports Medicine
200 Lakeville Road
Great Neck, New York 11021

Juan Wilson, M.D.
1900 Hempstead Turnpike
East Meadows, New York

OHIO

Josephine Aronica, M.D.
1867 W. Market Street
Akron, Ohio 44313

John M. Baron, D.O.
3101 Euclid Avenue, #201
Cleveland, Ohio 44115

James Dambrogio, D.O.
212 N. Main Street
Hubbard, Ohio 44425

James P. Frackelton, M.D.
24700 Center Ridge Road
Cleveland, Ohio 44145

David D. Goldberg, D.O.
4444 N. Main Street
Dayton, Ohio 45405

Jack E. Slingluff, D.O.
5850 Fulton Road, N.W.
Canton, Ohio 44718

Harold J. Wilson, M.D.
28 West Henderson Road
Columbus, Ohio 43214

OKLAHOMA

Leon Anderson, D.O.
121 South Second
Jenks, Oklahoma 74037

Charles H. Farr, M.D., Ph.D.
1312 N.W.—12th. Street
Suite 108
Moore, Oklahoma 73170

Larry L. Lowery, M.D.
Box 1590
Guymon, Oklahoma 73942

PENNSYLVANIA

Harold Buttram, M.D.
RD #3 Clymer Road
Quakertown, Pennsylvania 18951

Francis J. Cinelli, D.O.
153 N. 11th. Street
Bangor, Pennsylvania 18013

Lloyd Grumbles, M.D.
1601 Walnut Street
Suite B23
Philadelphia, Pennsylvania 19103

Arthur L. Koch, D.O.
337 E. Dia Avenue
Hazleton, Pennsylvania 18201

James S. Lapcevic, D.O., Ph.D.
129 E. Pine Street
Grove City, Pennsylvania 16127

Howard T. Lewis, M.D.
1241 Peermont Avenue
Pittsburgh, Pennsylvania 15216

Conrad G. Maulfair, D.O.
Main Street
Mertztown, Pennsylvania 19539

Milan J. Packovich, M.D.
2601—Fifth
McKeesport, Pennsylvania 15132

TENNESSEE

Donald C. Thompson, M.D.
828 West 4th. North Street
Morristown, Tennessee 37814

TEXAS

Jim P. Archer, D.O.
5202 Weber Road
Corpus Christi, Texas 78411

Ruben Berlanga, M.D.
580 Main Building
Houston, Texas 77002

Ann Bhuket, M.D.
1005—18th Street
Plano, Texas 75074

Richard O. Brennan, M.D.
5615 Richmond Avenue
Suite 151
Houston, Texas 77057

Herbert Carr, D.O.
P.O. Box 1179
Alamo, Texas 78516

William W. Halcomb, D.O.
8311 Shoal Creek Blvd.
Austin, Texas 78758

Paul McGuff, M.D.
3838 Hillcroft Street #312
Houston, Texas 77057

Gerald M. Parker, D.O.
4714 So. Western
Amarillo, Texas 79109

John Sessions, D.O.
1609 S. Margaret Street
Kirbyville, Texas 75956

John T. Taylor, D.O.
4714 S. Western
Amarillo, Texas 79109

J. Robert Winslow, D.O.
2745 Valwood Parkway
Dallas, Texas 75234

UTAH

Robert Vance, D.O.
5282 So. 320 West Suite D120
Salt Lake City, Utah 84107

VIRGINIA

Elmer Cranton, M.D.
Ripshin Road, P.O. Box 44
Trout Dale, Virginia 24378

Thomas J. Roberts, M.D.
31 West Loudoun Street
Leesburg, Virginia 22075

WASHINGTON

Murray L. Black, D.O.
622 S.—36th. Avenue
Yakima, Washington 98902

Leo Bolles, M.D.
15611 Bellevue-Redmond Road
Bellevue, Washington 98008

Jonathan Collin, M.D.
15611 Bellevue-Redmond Road
Bellevue, Washington 98008

Robert F. Kerr, M.D.
15613—Bel Red Road
Bellevue, Washington 98008

Quentin G.R. Schwenke, M.D.
321 Wellington
Walla Walla, Washington 99362

WASHINGTON D.C.

Howard Lutz M.D.
2139 Wisconsin Avenue N.W.
Suite 400
Washington, D.C. 20007

George Mitchell, M.D.
3201 New Mexico Avenue N.W.
Suite 230
Washington, D.C. 20016

WISCONSIN

Robert R. Stocker, D.O.
1005 N. Lake Road
Oconomowoc, Wisconsin 53066

NEW ZEALAND

Bruce A.J. Dewe, M.D.
Homestead Motel Clinic
Flaxmill Bay
Paradise Coast
Whitianga, New Zealand 2856

WEST GERMANY

Claus Martin, M.D.
The Four Seasons Clinic
and Health Resort
8183 Rottach—Egern, Faerberweg 3
West Germany 8183

Sustaining Exhibitors

The Key Company
734 North Harrison
St. Louis, Missouri 63122

The McGuff Company
3629 West MacArthur #202
Santa Ana, California 92704

Merit Pharmaceuticals
2622 Humboldt
Los Angeles, California 90031

Miller Pharmacal Group
Miller Pharmacal West
P.O. Box #279
West Chicago, Illinois 60185

Natural Scientifics
14018 North 49th. Street
Scottsdale, Arizona 85254

OCI Dietary Products
624 North Victory
Burbank, California 91502

Phyne Pharmaceuticals
5121 S.W. 90th. Avenue
Cooper City, Florida 33328

Vitaline Formulas
P.O. Box 6757
Incline Village, Nevada 89450

Index